LESS MEDICINE, MORE HEALTH

LESS MEDICINE, MORE HEALTH

7 ASSUMPTIONS THAT DRIVE TOO MUCH MEDICAL CARE

DR. H. GILBERT WELCH

BEACON PRESS
BOSTON

BEACON PRESS
Boston, Massachusetts
www.beacon.org

Beacon Press books
are published under the auspices of
the Unitarian Universalist Association of Congregations.

18   8 7 6 5 4

This book is printed on acid-free paper that meets the uncoated paper
ANSI/NISO specifications for permanence as revised in 1992.

Text design and composition by Kim Arney

Library of Congress Cataloging-in-Publication Data
Welch, H. Gilbert.
    Less medicine, more health : 7 assumptions that drive too much
medical care / Dr. H. Gilbert Welch.
        pages   cm
    Includes bibliographical references and index.
    ISBN 978-0-8070-7758-0 (paperback)
    ISBN 978-0-8070-7165-6 (ebook)
1. Health risk assessment. 2. Medicare. I. Title.
    RA427.3.W45 2015
    362.1—dc23

                                    2014031802

To patients everywhere

CONTENTS

INTRODUCTION

Our enthusiasm for everything medical

I AM THINKING ABOUT getting a brain transplant.

The technology is not quite there yet, but it's coming. I happen to know this because a friend of mine is a neuropsychiatric-cognitive surgeon—one of three in the nation. (Note: the denominator here is the number of similarly trained specialists, not the number of my friends.)

I've been talking to Haddad about my neuropsychiatric-cognitive problems. I used to be able to get up at three o'clock in the morning and catch up on work. Now I can't. I used to be carefree. Now I'm not. I used to be able to manage multiple tasks at the same time. Now if there are too many windows open on my computer, I have to close some. I used to be able to remember all my PINs and passwords. Now I can't.

I've never been able to remember people's names. While we're at it, I'd like that fixed too.

Haddad says a brain transplant will fix all this. He said it would be like increasing your RAM, processor, and hard drive—all at the same time. He also mentioned it would enhance my synaptic plasticity.

That sounds good. I'd like to have more plastic synapses. I'd like a new brain.

And I know I should probably do it sooner rather than later. I don't want to let my problems get too far advanced. What's the use of a new brain that's highly functioning, and without a care in the world, if the rest of my body can't enjoy it?

I figure the procedure will also have a beneficial side effect: it will lower my risk of brain cancer. I've been worrying about this a lot lately, ever since I heard that some academic medical centers are encouraging more "brain cancer awareness"—and offering free MRIs to screen for it. I've been surfing the net and have become aware that my risk of a brain tumor increases as I age.

So here's how I put it together: the donor brain will be presumably younger than mine, so my risk of brain cancer should be lowered. I understand there are some technical barriers to overcome. Hooking up the blood supply should be easy—it's basically a plumbing problem. Hooking up the spinal cord and the twelve cranial nerves will be more challenging. Haddad is working with a nerve stimulating factor to encourage these connections now. He says the trick is getting the connections right. I agree. I don't want to start talking and then put my foot in my mouth (although this already happens now).

For those of you who share my problems, I empathize. For those of you who thought this was going to be a nonfiction book, I apologize. The foregoing story exists only in my imagination; subsequent ones will be the real deal (although names, geography, and other potential identifying information may be altered).

And for those of you who think it all sounds far-fetched, consider the recent federal investment to map neurologic activity, the Brain Research through Advancing Innovative Neurotechnologies, or BRAIN for short. It has been thought of as an analogue of the Human Genome Project. Instead of mapping the genome, the initiative proposes to map the brain, and will undoubtedly feature some way-cool color images of brain activity. (They were going to call it the Brain Activity Map—until someone recognized the BAM acronym might be a problem. . . .) Whatever it is called, is there anyone who can't imagine that this effort will lead us to read something about the immense value of brain mapping? Not to mention some creative advertising copy?

Feeling down? Find out why and feel better—Get your brain mapped.

Having trouble remembering things? Your wires may be crossed—Get your brain mapped.

Unable to think clearly? Maybe your friends were right: you ought to have your head examined—Get your brain mapped.

And who can't imagine that there will be a subsequent "medical breakthrough"? Some drug, stimulator, implantable device, or even a surgical procedure that will make the map right. And who can't imagine that many of us may want to give one of these breakthroughs a try? (Whether the term "breakthrough" will be warranted is a separate question.)

■   ■   ■

WE AMERICANS CONSUME A LOT of medical care. By some metrics, we are the most medicalized society in the world. To be sure, there is an increasing amount of competition on this front as more and more of the developed world gives us a run for our money.

You might think that the biggest problem in medical care is that it costs too much. Or that health insurance is too expensive, too uneven, too complicated—and gives you too many forms to fill out. But the central problem is that too much medical care has too little value.

That's right, there can be too much medical care. Obviously this is not a problem for everyone, and it certainly isn't meant to deny that some people get too little medical care. But there has been a growing recognition that the conventional concern about "too little" needs to be balanced with a concern about "too much."

In a recent national survey of primary care physicians published by *Archives of Internal Medicine*, nearly one-half said their patients received too much medical care. Don't miss the fact that's the *doctors* talking.

Can you imagine the dentists saying that? Or the small animal vets?

And too much is not simply meant to imply wasteful care, but also harmful care.

I've been trying to raise physician consciousness about this problem for years. But some doctors don't need their consciousness raised—they know the problem better than I. After giving medical grand rounds at the University of Cincinnati, one came up to tell me a story. Not about one of his patients, but about his father.

Mr. Nadeau was eighty-five and in excellent health. He went to see his doctor simply for a routine checkup. The doctor performed a careful physical exam. Everything looked good, except for a bulge he thought he felt in Mr. Nadeau's belly—a bulge that might be an abdominal aortic aneurysm. An aneurysm is a ballooning of a blood vessel. As the blood vessel balloons, the vessel wall stretches, thins, and can rupture. The aorta is the largest blood vessel in the body. It originates in the heart, travels upwards in the chest (to supply blood to the head and arms), and then curves downwards into the abdomen (to supply blood to the digestive tract, kidneys, and legs). A ruptured abdominal aorta can cause massive blood loss and sudden death. That's worrisome.

So the doctor ordered an abdominal ultrasound, the same technology used to show expectant mothers their baby. The ultrasound showed that Mr. Nadeau's aorta was normal—there was no abdominal aortic aneurysm. But the ultrasound found something else to worry about. It found something abnormal on Mr. Nadeau's pancreas. The radiologist thought it was a small growth. It had nothing to do with what the doctor felt on the physical exam; it was way too small to be felt. But it still could be cancer.

She recommended a CT scan of the abdomen, an exam that combines X-rays and computing power to produce a more detailed picture than ultrasound. The CT scan showed the pancreas was normal.

But the CT scan found something else to worry about. It found a nodule on Mr. Nadeau's liver. The radiologist recommended a liver biopsy to see what the nodule was (it could be cancer too). To biopsy a liver nodule a gastroenterologist inserts a needle through the skin, through the liver, and into the nodule. To cut out a piece of tissue big enough for a pathologist to examine under a microscope, the gastroenterologist has to use a good-sized needle, roughly the caliber of a small knitting needle.

The pathologic diagnosis was hemangioma, a benign growth made up of lots of blood vessels. Given that a small knitting needle was cutting through a growth full of blood vessels, you won't be surprised by what happened next.

Bleeding. Mr. Nadeau was in the hospital for a week. He needed about ten units of blood (his physician son had a hard time keeping count). He was in a lot of pain and was given morphine. Once patients are on pain medications and bedridden in the hospital, other things happen. Mr. Nadeau was no exception: he became unable to pee. He had to have a urinary catheter put in. It was an ordeal. Although Mr. Nadeau did not die, he could have.

That's too much medicine.

It's tempting to look for someone to blame here—someone who has made a mistake. Maybe the gastroenterologist should have decided to watch the nodule, instead of biopsying it. Maybe the radiologist should have recognized that the nodule was a hemangioma. Maybe the primary care doctor should not have examined Mr. Nadeau's abdomen. Maybe Mr. Nadeau should not have gone in for a checkup in the first place.

Or maybe all of us should reconsider our assumptions and expectations for medical care.

If you wonder whether Mr. Nadeau's story of harmful medical care is one of a kind, I suggest you see a doctor. Ask him or her. I bet you'll hear another story.

Too many people are being made to worry about diseases they don't have and are at only average risk to get. You may not consider that a harm, but remember health is not simply a state of physical being—it's also a state of mind.

Too many people are being tested and exposed to the harmful effects of the testing process: the anxiety of false alarms and the vulnerability caused by ambiguous findings (*"you don't have the disease, but you aren't normal"*). Not to mention the complications of diagnostic procedures.

Too many people are being treated with treatments they don't need or can't benefit from. Treatment interventions can have substantial physical harms such as medication reactions, surgical complications, even death.

How did we get here?

The doctors' standard answer to the question is: lawyers. We call it defensive medicine. Fear of malpractice does influence our behavior, but it's clearly not the whole story. I ask my colleagues who blame lawyers to consider this thought experiment: Would the problems of overuse simply disappear if the lawyers simply disappeared? That tends to help them understand that a myriad of forces are at play.

The economists' standard answer to the question is (surprise) economics. Here's how they see it: physicians are paid more to do more, and insurance, not the patient, foots most of the bill. Paying physicians a fee every time they provide a service encourages them to order more tests and procedures. Because patients are shielded from the cost by a third party (the insurer), they have little incentive to scrutinize the value of the services. In other words, economists see the combination of fee for service and third-party payment as a powerful recipe for too much care.

I think of it as the free food problem. In my younger days, hospitals routinely gave doctors in training, even lowly medical students, free food. Not that it was that good; this was the era when the term "hospital food" was right up there with "school lunch." But it was free. Instead of deciding between two entrees, I just got both. And I'd eat both. Plus, since somewhere in the hospital there always seemed to be a staff member having a birthday, I could always manage to find free dessert at a nursing station.

Now my problem is at medical conferences. To be sure, the food has gotten healthier—less fat, less sugar, less processed—but it's still free (more precisely, wrapped into the registration fee). But the end result is the same. I eat too much.

And don't get me started on "all you can eat" buffets.

Note that the free food problem exists even without the fee for service incentive. Imagine free food *and* paying food-service workers more to put more food on your plate. *Can you say gluttony?* So the economists have a point: incentives matter. But there is a wrinkle. You can't just grab some medical care to go. It takes time—and can have some annoying qualities. Plus it generally doesn't taste that good. So the source of too much medical care must be more complicated than free food.

The recipe of adding fee for service to third-party payment to cook up too much medical care would not work without strong underlying beliefs about the value of the product. The general public harbors assumptions about medical care that encourage overuse. Assumptions like: it's always better to fix the problem, sooner (or newer) is always better, or it never hurts to get more information.

I'm not blaming the public; many of these assumptions flow directly from information provided to them, be it from the news media, talk shows, advertising, PR campaigns, disease advocacy groups, public service announcements, or doctors themselves.

Regardless of their source, these assumptions lead individuals to have an excessively optimistic view of medical care. That leads them to seek—some would say to demand, others to accept—too much care. These assumptions also drive public policy in the same direction, to our detriment.

A growing number of doctors understand that the prevailing assumptions drive too much medical care. Some of them have contributed to this book through their writing and research. And while more and more doctors recognize that these assumptions are erroneous, they still assume it's what their patients assume, and so they act accordingly. The truth is that doctors find it's much harder to challenge the assumptions than to go with the flow.

This book is about challenging these assumptions—and helping us all avoid too much medical care.

■   ■   ■

I'M A PRIMARY CARE PHYSICIAN. My specialty certification is in internal medicine, but my perspective is more aligned with family practice. I did a rotating internship, with pediatrics, obstetrics, surgery, and medicine. I worked as a general medical officer for the US Public Health Service in Bethel, Alaska (unbelievably, I was the surgical officer). I've held a range of temporary duty posts, from being a ship's physician for the NOAA ship *Oceanographer* (from Townsville, Australia, to Seattle, Washington) to covering the National Health Service Corps site in the coalfields of western Virginia (the part of Virginia that is west of West Virginia). As a clinician, I have been more drawn to small, isolated rural hospitals than to large, academic medical centers. That's why I've spent the last twenty-some years as an outpatient doctor for the VA hospital in White River Junction, Vermont.

Although I spend less and less time seeing patients with each successive year (and may have stopped by the time you are reading this), I'm drawn to common medical problems and the big picture. I like medicine and believe it can do really good things for people. And I like people. It's the bad things medicine can do to people that I don't like.

I'm a health services researcher; some might call me a medical care epidemiologist. That means I am interested in patterns of medical care, across both time and place. It's why I came to Dartmouth—it is a great place to do this kind of work. My research career has largely focused on the problems created by early diagnosis, particularly cancer screening.

Finally, I'm a classroom teacher. Before I went to medical school, I was a high school math teacher. Soon after I joined the Dartmouth Medical School faculty, I was asked to teach statistics. Over the past two decades my charge has expanded to include epidemiology, study design, and health policy. My student population has expanded as well; it now includes Dartmouth undergraduates, public health students, medical students, and mid-career professionals.

This book reflects my experience from each of these three jobs. But the idea really came from my work in the classroom, and the advice given me by a business school dean.

A business school dean?

A few years ago, Dartmouth got a new president. He wanted to build a new science, what he called the science of health care delivery. His approach was to bring together two very different cultures at Dartmouth: the Dartmouth Institute for Health Policy and Clinical Practice (that's the shop that has been asking hard questions about US medical care for over a quarter century, produces the *Dartmouth Atlas*, and is my employer), and the Amos Tuck School of Business (that's the first graduate school of management ever established—a bold move by Dartmouth in 1900—and one now consistently ranked among the top MBA programs). The vehicle to bring these two cultures together was a program to teach mid-career health care executives how to better manage health care. It was directed by the senior associate dean of Tuck, Bob Hansen.

I was more than a little skeptical when I first met Bob (come on, he's a business school guy). Turns out he's from the UP, that cool peninsula off Wisconsin, just south of Lake Superior, that for some reason belongs to Michigan. That was intriguing (I told you I was drawn to isolated regions). More intriguing was that Bob didn't want me just to teach what I usually did: statistics and study design. He had read some of my research and some of my efforts to communicate with the general public. He wanted me to get the students to think differently about medical care, to dig into prevailing assumptions and reveal what he dubbed the disturbing truths. I'm sure he was partly driven by marketing (come on, he's a business school guy). Nevertheless, it was a good call.

There are more assumptions (and disturbing truths) than appear here. This book is focused on those assumptions that are widely shared by patients and their families. So erroneous assumptions made by doctors, such as "malpractice is the only driver of health care costs," and by policymakers, like "quality metrics reliably measure quality," won't appear here.

The book may encourage you to think more critically about medical care—more critically than most people do. I do not expect (nor want) you to agree with everything I say. Let's be clear: medical decisions are not simply about science; they also involve value judgments. But if you get through the book, my bet is many of you will see my basic point: as a society, we have overstated the benefits of medical care and underplayed its harms. And that it is just possible less medicine would be better for our health.

I hope physicians will share this book with their patients, particularly those who want to understand why less medical care might actually be better for them. Full disclosure: there could be some tough sledding ahead—some anatomy, physiology, epidemiology, medical research, and clinical medicine. All of these fields are important to get a feel for what really goes on in the practice of medicine.

Conversely, I also hope patients will share this book with their doctors. Perhaps your doctor already gets the big picture; perhaps not. Either way, a little nudge from patients may help more physicians do the right thing.

I believe questioning assumptions about the value of medical care is the key ingredient for a more sustainable health care system. If the word "sustainable" makes you gag, go with "more affordable" or "taking fewer resources from other important social goods" or "not impoverishing our children and our children's children." More importantly, I believe that questioning medical care assumptions is an important element in promoting healthier expectations and a healthier population.

That's right, the solution to the cost conundrum, and the road to health itself, is to have all Americans, all western Europeans, and, hell, the whole world buy (and read) this book.

Oops. Am I starting to sound like a used-car salesman . . . ?

So let's deal with the elephant in the room. A few of my critics have suggested that I'm just trying to sell books. Here's an e-mail I got from an orthopedic surgeon in Florida (after I had an op-ed published in the *New York Times*):

> How is it possible that such an educated man can be so naive about our
> medical system? Your writings serve no purpose other than to insight
> a furor in the general public and likely earn you more monies in roy-
> alties for your books.

OK. It should have been "incite," not "insight," but cut him a break. You get the criticism. And it's a reasonable concern. In my profession, I regret to say, it is always reasonable to worry about financial interests. Medicine has been increasingly dominated by the interest of making money. Too many doctors seem to view the medical profession less as a calling—and more as an investment opportunity. Some routinely serve as consultants to drug companies and device manufacturers (some consult for multiple companies at the same time). There are other opportunities as well, like forming new biotech companies, serving on speaker bureaus, and writing books.

All the royalties for this book will go to charity. I'm not referring to the broad IRS definition of charity, which includes donations to causes that only concern affluent people like myself (like donating to my alma mater or to help conserve land next to my house). Instead I mean what my parents meant when they used the word *charity*: an effort to help people truly in need. Specifically the royalties will go to local charities in the Upper Connecticut Valley of New Hampshire and Vermont, organizations that repair old housing, provide shelter, recapture and distribute food, and help the poor with unexpected bills, like a major car repair so that they can get to work or like another fuel oil delivery so they can get through the northern New England winter.

This is not in reaction to my critics; it's my standard operating procedure. All the royalties on my prior two books (*Should I Be Tested for Cancer?* and *Overdiagnosed: Making People Sick in the Pursuit of Health*) went to these charities.

Until recently, I haven't been comfortable making this public. I'm not sure I can articulate exactly why—it's something about not wanting to project myself as being "holier than thou" (which I'm most definitely not, ask my high school buddies—Eee, JB, K-dog, and the M.A.N.—they'll provide plenty of counterexamples). Plus I didn't want to give the impression that I thought there is something wrong with authors making money on books—there's not. For many, it is their main source of income.

But I have a job, one that I'm well remunerated for. In fact, in my first contact with an agent over ten years ago, I got this advice: "Keep your day job" (not that I was seriously considering changing jobs). I have the luxury of being able to live off my salary. More importantly, I didn't want to be profiting from what I knew would be a controversial and disturbing message.

I wanted to write this book to help people have healthier expectations for medical care. Medical care is neither a catastrophe waiting to happen, nor is it a panacea. Because most people err toward the latter view, here I focus on what can go wrong. And I'll give you a few simple strategies, which I'll call prescriptions, to avoid too much medical care.

■ ■ ■

BEING CLEAR ABOUT WHAT can go wrong can be disturbing. I don't relish disturbing people. One of my radiology friends, a doctor who reads mammograms, recently lamented that I was scaring women away from being screened. That hurt. (I wasn't quick enough to point out that his colleagues have been scaring women *into* being screened for over thirty years, but that's a story for later.)

I don't want to scare you, but I do want to make sure you get both sides of the story. You are undoubtedly familiar with the word *medical* being juxtaposed with the word *miracle* or *breakthrough*. You have been taught that medical care is the path to health. You have been told to "see your doctor." To have a more balanced view of medical care requires some attention to the other side of the story. But I don't want you to be so disturbed that you avoid medical care entirely.

There is a lot of good in medical care, particularly in the care of the acutely ill and injured. I was reminded of this fact as I began writing this book. My wife had spent the entire hot, muggy July day outside fencing (meaning with posts, not swords). It cooled off that evening, but she still felt hot. I wrote it off to a touch of heat stroke. Demonstrating highly unusual behavior, Linda spent the better part of the next day in bed. When I got home, she was hotter and sicker. We dusted off my mother's glass thermometer—the one not infrequently popped into my mouth when I wanted to avoid school (the one that never seemed to read high enough)—and took her temperature. It was 103.6. For an adult, that's an impressive fever.

Linda's temperature was lower the next morning and she went to see a doctor who wasn't her husband. Her temperature was nearly normal in clinic. Typical—go to the doctor and the problem goes away. The doctor suggested that the fever was likely due to a viral infection, she would probably get better, and the best course of action was to watch and wait. (For the record, this is exactly what I would have done, but I was more than happy to have the decision on somebody else's shoulders. . . .)

It was another hot sunny day. And Linda's car had been sitting in the sun for a couple of hours with the windows up. According to a Stanford study of "enclosed vehicles," that means the car's internal temperature was somewhere between 120 and 140 degrees. Oh, and the air conditioner hadn't worked for months. (Not that this had been a concern for months, because in Vermont the heater is far more relevant for most of the year.) Linda drove the fifteen miles home without opening the windows. In medicine, that's what we call a "salient" piece of clinical history. The reason she hadn't opened the windows of the 120-plus degree car was that she felt cold. That means she was in the process of developing one hell of a fever. She took her temperature again. It was 103.6 again. She called the doctor. The doctor was impressed.

Linda sent me an e-mail at work. The subject line read, "Please come home." In twenty-five-plus years of marriage, I'd never seen that before. I was impressed.

She was sick—as sick as I have ever seen her. She had a high fever and was having trouble thinking and speaking (that's usually my department, not hers). I was worried. But the medical care system did exactly what we would all want it to do. It kicked in. The doctor got blood cultures, a complete blood count, and liver function tests. Linda's white count was much lower than normal, her platelet count had dropped, and she had signs of hepatitis. That told me Linda was sick, and it wasn't from the standard bacterial causes I would normally consider, such as a urinary tract infection, a pneumonia, or an abdominal infection.

But once again, Linda's primary care doctor did exactly what I would have done—seek help. And, in this case, the relevant help came in the form of a physician trained in infectious disease. Turns out acute intermittent fever, low white count, low platelet count, mild hepatitis, and no rash—in an adult who spends a large portion of her time outside in our part of the country—is pretty good history for a rare tick-borne infection: human granulocytic anaplasmosis. Rare as in, according to the Centers for Disease Control, six cases per million people.

There was no way I was going to make that diagnosis. Nor would most primary care doctors, unless they had happened to have already seen a case of human granulocytic anaplasmosis.

The good news is that the infection is readily treatable with an antibiotic that has been around since the late 1960s, doxycycline. Linda was a lot better in twenty-four hours, and fully recovered a week later.

To me this is an example of medical care at its best. You have the misfortune of having something go acutely wrong. You have prompt access to a caring, engaged, competent primary care practitioner. If it turns out your problem is a rare one, your primary care practitioner has ready access to expert help.

When I think about what I most want out of my medical care system, my first priority is to have a system that excels in the care and treatment of the acutely ill and injured. If I develop an acute febrile illness—or have a heart attack or develop intestinal/urinary obstruction or get hurt in a car or bike accident—I will eagerly seek medical care.

This is the most important part of medical care, but it's not what most of medical care is. And much of medical care doesn't reliably lead to better health.

ALL RISKS CAN BE LOWERED

Disturbing truth: Risks can't always be
lowered—and trying creates risks of its own

I HAVE A STUNNING admission for a doctor to make: I am overweight.

Seriously. Not seriously overweight, instead I am being serious when I say I am overweight. As of this morning, my BMI—body mass index—was 25.4. According to the National Heart, Lung, and Blood Institute, everyone with a BMI of 25 or above is overweight. And they are clear that this isn't just a cosmetic problem (that's good, because I've got plenty of other cosmetic problems to worry about anyway). Being overweight is a condition that "greatly raises" my risk of heart attack, heart failure, stroke, diabetes, and cancer. I bet it's a genetic disorder— my mom was overweight.

I'm sure you're thinking, "What a tragedy." But don't worry, by my estimation well over half of the Supreme Court is overweight. They seem to be doing fine.

Then again, I could undoubtedly find some cigarette smokers without lung cancer or heart disease. Would that mean smoking doesn't cause the diseases?

We are subjected to a confusing barrage of information about dangers to our health. Is sunlight something to be feared as a cause of cancer—or something to be sought out as a way to produce vitamin D? Does wine raise your risk of breast cancer—or lower your risk of heart disease? Do cell phones cause brain cancer—or are their allegedly harmful electromagnetic fields actually therapeutic? Does chocolate lower your risk of stroke—or raise your risk of heartburn, cavities, weight gain, and diabetes? Should I worry more about the dangers of getting too much of these things—or too little?

There is so much noise, so much attention to reports about trivial or nonexistent risks, that I sometimes imagine it's all some conspiracy intended to distract us from the signal—things that really do matter. But the much more likely explanation is this: the topic of health risks is one that helps sell magazines, or teases viewers into watching the evening news, or drives people to websites—and, in turn, helps sell medical care.

Even the word *risk* is confusing. Historically, the word refers to the possibility of loss, injury, or other adverse or unwelcome circumstance. In finance, it refers to the chance you will lose money. In statistics, it simply refers to the probability of some uncertain future event. But when it comes to human health, the idea of possibility, chance, or probability typically gets lost and a risk becomes a threat—a threat that must be dealt with by medical care.

All health risks are not equal. Some are real; others may not even exist. Some are really important; others are overstated. And while it would seem that trying to lower real, important health risks would always make sense, it turns out that trying can create risks of its own.

SIGNAL: RISKS THAT MATTER

A few years ago I had the privilege of speaking to the Montana Medical Association in the state's capitol. I drove into Helena from the east, through high plains above the Missouri River rimmed by mountains—it's beautiful country. Lewis and Clark explored the area in 1805 and, because Clark managed to get a number of cactus spines in his feet, he named the nearby creek and surrounding valley Prickly Pear.

Just off the road, there was an old homestead and a historic marker. I had to check it out. The marker was the classic western standard: a massive piece of wood, painted brown, with carved letters, painted white. It identified the site as the homestead of Jonathon and Elmira Manlove, who, along with their two small children, were the first permanent settlers in the Prickly Pear Valley.

As I walked over to explore the structure, I looked back at the sign and saw something totally unexpected: it had been reused. The flipside of the sign had similar lettering, although the paint had faded considerably.

Written in the 1950s, it reflected the boosterism often associated with American small towns. It made sure visitors to the town that grew up along Prickly Pear Creek—East Helena—were aware just how prominent its three major employers were at the time.

The American Smelting and Refining Company produces lead bullion from ores shipped in from Idaho, Montana, Newfoundland, Canada, South America and Australia.

The Anaconda Company produces zinc oxide from the slag of American Smelting and Refining.

The American Chemet plant in East Helena processes leaded zinc products and Montana talc for use as paint pigments and in the manufacture of Columbia Paints.

It also offered this warm invitation for visitors:

The city park is here for your enjoyment with tables, benches, rest rooms, wading pool and playground equipment.

I doubt you'll see many signs like this anymore. The juxtaposition of lead paint and playground equipment—or, for that matter, heavy metals and wading pools—just doesn't project the image of a desirable community these days. Particularly when you can turn around and view massive piles of contaminated slag next to Prickly Pear Creek. It became one of the nation's first Superfund sites over thirty years ago.

Lead was among the first known environmental hazards. Its toxicity was recognized in Greco-Roman times and was a frequent topic in the medical literature of the 1800s. Historically, exposure involved drinking (water from leaded pipes, moonshine from leaded stills); more recently, inhalation (leaded gasoline fumes) and ingestion (peeling leaded paint). Acute poisoning is dramatic, with headaches, seizures, loss of vision, paralysis, and death. Chronic poisoning is more subtle but still obvious: it could be seen in the skin, on the teeth and gums, under the microscope in red blood cells, and—with the advent of X-rays—on the bones. Chronic lead poisoning is now recognized to have profound effects on cognition, adversely affecting intelligence and behavior. You get the picture—lead is bad for you.

So it's tempting to mock the town boosters of Montana in the 1950s. But before you do, you should know something about the physicians of Massachusetts in the 1950s: most were cigarette smokers. To be clear, there is no reason to believe there was anything peculiar about the physicians of Massachusetts—except the fact that one of them took the initiative to survey his colleagues about their smoking habits in 1954. Throughout the world, doctors were smoking.

In fact, arguably the single most important piece of evidence that cigarette smoking causes lung cancer came from observations of British physicians who smoked. Starting in the early 1900s, a rapid rise in lung cancer deaths was noted throughout the developed world, in Australia, Britain, Canada, Denmark, Japan, Switzerland, Turkey, and the United States. Although some of the increase was believed to be the result of better reporting practices, its magnitude—over tenfold among British males—demanded that other causes be considered. The widespread increase in tobacco smoking was a leading hypothesis but not the only one.

For the past fifteen years I have related this story to introduce epidemiology—the science of the patterns and causes of disease—to medical students, public health students, and undergraduates. I always ask them to guess what the major competing hypothesis was. Few guess right: the general decline in atmospheric quality.

Part of the reason is surely because the case against cigarette smoking is now so obviously closed. However, it certainly wasn't closed at the time. When Massachusetts physicians were asked in 1954 whether they agreed with the statement "Heavy smoking may lead to lung cancer," about a third said no—even with the "may" in there. But I think another part of the reason students can't guess the competing hypothesis is that they have little inkling about just how bad air pollution was.

It's tempting to think of our current environment as being horribly degraded, a potent threat to our health. But here historical context is relevant. In the middle of the twentieth century, urban air quality was much worse than today. Pittsburgh was the poster child for the problem: the confluence of two tight river valleys, full of steel mills and a sooty downtown that featured darkness at noon. If you want to see it, I recommend the Smoke Control Lantern Slide Collection recently posted by the University of Pittsburgh. But it wasn't just Pittsburgh and steel mills; it was industrialization, and sulfur from coal burning in particular, that produced bad air throughout the developed world. When bad air stagnated over cities there were immediate health effects: people died, especially those who already had heart and lung problems. "Killer smogs" led to the deaths of tens of people in nearby Donora, Pennsylvania, in 1948, hundreds in New York City in 1953, and thousands in London that same year.

Suffice it to say that degraded atmospheric quality was a plausible explanation for the epidemic of lung cancer. But it wasn't the right one.

Sorting out competing explanations for outbreaks of disease is what epidemiology is all about. Classically, epidemiology examines exposures relevant to infectious disease, from water supplies as the source of cholera epidemics in the mid-1800s to food supplies as the source of recent salmonella outbreaks. In the mid-1900s epidemiology began to tackle exposures relevant to chronic disease, and explaining the epidemic of lung cancer was an important place to start. If you ask epidemiologists whom to credit for this evolution from infectious to chronic disease—as well as for closing the case on cigarette smoking and turning their field into a rigorous science—they'll all respond with the same two Englishmen, Doll and Hill.

Sir Richard Doll and Sir Austin Bradford Hill (of course, the Queen didn't knight them till years later) had concerned themselves with lung cancer epidemics for a while. In 1950 they published what was one of the first case-control studies, in which they compared the smoking history of patients admitted to London hospitals with lung cancer (the cases), with age- and sex-matched patients admitted to the same hospitals, at about the same time but who had other diagnoses (the controls). The lung cancer patients were much more likely to have been smokers, but the new study design was undoubtedly confusing, and not that convincing, to physicians.

Then Doll and Hill had a stroke of genius: study physicians themselves. Like most great ideas, it was conceptually simple. In 1951, they sent out a short questionnaire to British physicians, asking a few questions about their use of tobacco. Approximately 34,000 males and 6,000 females responded. Then they waited four years to find out who had died, and why.

What was the genius in studying physicians? Tactically, it was a perfect population to study given Doll and Hill's interest in convincing physicians themselves about the dangers of cigarette smoking. Perhaps more important, however, was that this study population also provided a practical advantage. Keeping track of forty thousand people for four years is not an easy task for two investigators (particularly without the help of Facebook or LinkedIn). People move around. But British doctors were already being tracked, by two groups no less—the National Health Service and the British Medical Association. They kept track of where doctors lived and when they died. All Doll and Hill needed were the death certificates to determine the cause of death.

There were approximately 1,700 deaths among the males and 100 among the females. The women didn't smoke enough—and didn't die enough—to provide much useful information.

Among the 34,000 male physicians, about 28,000 were smokers and 6,000 were not. In terms of smoking physicians, at least, the Brits beat the Yanks. During the four years of observation there were eighty-four males who died from lung cancer. Eighty-three were smokers; one was not.

Wow. I'll do the math for you. Eighty-three lung cancer deaths among 28,000 smokers (83/28,000), as compared to 1 death among 6,000 nonsmokers (1/6,000), produces a ratio of about 18:1. That means that British physicians who smoked were eighteen times more likely to die from lung cancer than nonsmokers. That got the doctors' attention.

Doll and Hill did much more with the data. They demonstrated that the more a doctor smoked, the more likely he was to die from lung cancer. Those smoking more than a pack a day were more than thirty times more likely than nonsmokers to die from lung cancer. They also showed that smoking was as bad for doctors living in the clean air of rural England as it was for doctors living in smog-filled London, which provided powerful evidence that their findings were not the result of air pollution. And Doll and Hill had yet another important finding: a doctor who had stopped smoking experienced a progressive decline in his risk of dying from lung cancer. Recent quitters, a little; long-ago quitters, a lot.

Lead and cigarettes represent very real, important health risks. Lead was easier to figure out, because its acute toxicity was obvious, and it has been easily measurable in both the environment and humans for years. And no one got lead poisoning without lead exposure. Cigarettes were a little tougher, since they produced no obvious acute problems, and the measurement of exposure had to be based on self-report. Adding to the challenge was the fact that some people do get lung cancer without ever having smoked. But Doll and Hill closed the case.

Lead and cigarettes are very real, important health risks that have been successfully lowered. Getting the lead out of gasoline and paint has been arguably the most important environmental intervention to protect human health. (Unless you want to count basic sanitation to protect drinking water as an environmental intervention, in which case you hold a trump card.) Smoking cessation has been undoubtedly the single most important behavioral intervention to protect human health.

NOISE: TRIVIAL OR NONEXISTENT RISKS

There has been a lot of chronic disease epidemiology since Doll and Hill. We've learned a lot more about the dangers of cigarette smoking— it's not just about lung cancer. Cigarette smoking also raises the risk of other cancers, heart disease, and lung disease. Because of the combined effect of all these diseases, regular smokers die at nearly double the rate of those who don't smoke. Chronic disease epidemiology has also taught us that asbestosis, radiation, and certain viruses cause cancer, and that high cholesterol and high blood pressure are important risk factors for heart disease. It has also taught us much about the relationship between diet, alcohol, exercise, income, education, social class, and human health.

But that's all old news.

What's the new news? At the time of this writing it's "Cancer Risk Increases with Height." Apparently for every four-inch increase in height, there is a 13 percent increase in the risk for developing cancer. At least, according to the journal *Cancer Epidemiology, Biomarkers, and Prevention*.

I couldn't make up a better example of noise. Give me a break. Full disclosure: not only am I overweight, I'm tall: 6 feet 4 inches tall. I'll spare you all the methodological questions that lead me to wonder whether this study is even right. Because even if it were right, I'd still have two big questions to ask:

So what? A 13 percent increase is tiny. Doesn't come close to doubling my risk—roughly the point I might start paying attention. For that to happen, I'd have to be taller than Shaq (or Yao Ming). A lot taller, as in about nine feet tall. Percentage increases tend to exaggerate effects: a doubling of risk is a 100 percent increase. Regular cigarette smoking increases the risk of lung cancer death by a factor of twenty to thirty—that's a 1,900 percent to 2,900 percent increase. So even if the study were right, height would have considerably less than 1 one-hundredth of that effect.

Now what? What should tall people do with this information? Run out and get a full body scan? Shrink? Stop wearing high heels? Make sure that their children are poorly nourished? Don't do that, because I also found an article titled "Short Stature Is Associated with Coronary Heart Disease." (You might think I'm making this stuff up, but I'm not.)

Welcome to the modern world of chronic disease epidemiology, where big data too often identifies tiny risks but produces unimportant information. It's a world where only the extremes of tiny get published and reported: coffee is either "definitely a little good" or "definitely a little bad" for you; it never has no effect at all.

Chronic disease epidemiology has hit the flat of the curve. Sure, there is always room to make some basic public health points—such as having a handgun in the house increases your chance of a handgun death, or driving slower decreases your chance of a motor vehicle death (whether these observations warrant legislation is a separate question, but there is little question that they represent important information for the public to know). But the big risks to human health have largely been identified, because they are relatively easy to detect. I'm confident we're not about to find another risk factor like cigarettes—the smoking guns are too obvious. Now, we have a small army of epidemiologists examining huge databases, looking for tiny effects. The tiny effects they find are often not the result of the postulated factor but of other factors that are unmeasured, or unmeasurable.

Then selective pressures come into play. Researchers communicate selectively: they are more likely to write up their finding of an effect, than their finding of no effect. The problem is compounded by medical journals that publish selectively, favoring studies with worrisome or protective findings over those that show no relationship at all. Finally, the media tops it all off with selective reporting, displaying much more interest in dramatic findings than mundane ones (like, coffee isn't worth worrying about).

And don't think the fact that many epidemiologists are being redeployed to genetics solves these problems. Because *genetic epidemiology* shares all of the same problems.

An epidemiologist for the American Cancer Society summed up the situation: "With epidemiology you can tell a little thing from a big thing. What's very hard to do is to tell a little thing from nothing at all." And that was almost fifteen years ago.

CHANCE HAPPENS

A few years back, a fascinating investigation was published on astrological signs and admission to the hospital. In case you weren't part of the Age of Aquarius and weren't subjected to the 5th Dimension's single over and over and over on your AM radio, the astrological signs are the twelve sectors of the ecliptic, starting at the vernal equinox. Depending on where the sun was in the zodiac the day you were born, you are either an Aries, Taurus, Gemini, Cancer, Leo, Virgo, Libra, Scorpio, Sagittarius, Capricorn, Aquarius, or Pisces.

I'm a Taurus—a bull. According to this investigation, those of us born between the 30th and 60th degree of the zodiac face a 27 percent above average risk to be hospitalized for diverticular disease. That's when little pouches bulge out of the colon, like a weak tire wall, and then get infected. Looks like I'm destined to get bowel problems.

And there's more. The investigators found that the risk for seventy-one other types of hospitalization was "significantly raised" simply by being born under a specific astrological sign. My personal favorite was that Scorpios—named after a predatory arthropod, a nasty bunch for sure—had a 57 percent increased risk of being hospitalized for abscesses of the anal and rectal region.

I know this is all beginning to sound like shit. Because it is.

But that was precisely the authors' point. Admittedly, their language was more eloquent than mine; their paper was titled "Testing Multiple Statistical Hypotheses Resulted in Spurious Associations."

They were using big data: five million hospital admissions in the Canadian province of Ontario. And they were demonstrating the problems with its use. The data included the reason for the hospitalization, which was categorized into one of 223 common diagnoses. The data also included the patients' date of birth, which was categorized into one of twelve astrological signs.

With 5 million admissions, 223 diagnoses, and 12 signs, of course they were bound to find a bunch of apparent relationships. Chance happens, particularly in big data. No one actually believes that your astrological sign is responsible for specific hospital diagnoses. OK, I'm sure someone does, but we don't believe him.

I'd like to think Sir Bradford Hill actually anticipated this problem in the 1950s. He certainly thought hard about the question of what constitutes cause and effect. He delineated a list of criteria that suggest a causal relationship is likely. That list has become known as the Hill criteria—one of which is that to argue that something is causal, it sure helps to have some plausible mechanism between the cause and effect.

Although he was clear that this criterion, now called biological plausibility, was imperfect ("What is biologically plausible depends upon the biological knowledge of the day"), it's a damn good starting point. Certainly producing smoke by burning finely cut, cured, acidified plant leaves (along with a bunch of other additives) and then inhaling it regularly into the lungs is a more biologically plausible cause of lung cancer than where the sun was in the zodiac the day you were born.

Hill's number-one criterion was that strong associations are more likely to represent cause and effect. A strong association is one that increases risk by tenfold or more (more than a 900 percent increase)—like regular cigarette smoking and lung cancer. A weak association is one that doesn't even double the risk (less than a 100 percent increase)—like those predatory Scorpios who were 80 percent more likely to be admitted for leukemia. Hill would have taken one look at that and declared, "That's not signal; that's noise." There is no perfect dividing line between strong and weak association. My rule of thumb is simply to ignore anything less than double—that is, ignore all those double digit percentage increases. That won't get rid of all the noise, but it will get rid of a lot.

FILTERING OUT NOISE—A PRIMER

Let me start by saying that experts, in any area, tend not to like rules of thumb. They can always imagine conditions under which the rule fails and they can always nominate other factors that are relevant to the decision. Epidemiologists are no exception. So it's tempting for me to say, "You need to take a course in epidemiology" or, more precisely, "You need to take *my* course in epidemiology." But that's too easy. I think we have an obligation to give the public some concrete guidance.

My use of the word *noise* actually combines two attributes: risks that do not exist in the first place and risks that are so small that they are unimportant, even if they do, in fact, exist. The rule of thumb is my crude attempt to deal with both.

The first question is *"Does the risk actually exist?"* In other words, is there truly a cause-effect relationship? Hill was arguing that strong associations are more likely to be real, while weak associations are more likely to be the result of some other factor. To address this question, many epidemiologists would argue for an even higher threshold: ignore anything that isn't at least a three- or fourfold increase. Doll even suggested that the lower limit of the margin of error (the 95 percent confidence interval) should be at least threefold to be persuasive. Of course other things come into play—the study design, the statistics, the biological plausibility, the collective evidence from other studies (did I mention you should take my course?)—but the strength of the association is central.

The second question is *"Assuming the cause-effect relationship does exist, is it big enough to pay attention to?"* This is again a function of the strength of the association, but it is also a function of where you start: the baseline risk. In other words, doubling your money has a very different connotation if you start with one dollar as opposed to one thousand. Thankfully, for the average person, most bad health events are rare: as in, occur to less than 1 percent of us in the next decade. Doubling that risk takes it to less than 2 percent. When considering probabilities like this, it's always useful to flip the frame: the chance of *not* having the event moves from 99 percent to 98 percent. That feels like noise. To be sure, a doubling of a more common health event might be more concerning.

Accept that any rule of thumb can be wrong—and in both directions. Pay attention to those things that double, triple, or increase your risk tenfold and ignore those stories that talk about "threats to your health" followed by double-digit percentage increases. Get rid of some noise.

One of my epidemiology mentors at the University of Washington summed up the noise problem this way in the journal *Science*. "[There are] just too many false alarms. When we do have a serious message, I fear it won't be heeded because of the large number of false messages." Crying wolf is certainly one problem, but what's worse is when we doctors do something based on false messages.

DO SOMETHING—UNEXPECTED CONSEQUENCES

My mother was quite a character. Trained as a nurse at the Yale-New Haven hospital during World War II, she left nursing to have three boys. In 1960 my family moved west as my father joined the faculty at the University of Colorado. Once settled in Boulder, Mom became vigorously engaged in battles on behalf of Planned Parenthood and population control.

When I was in high school, she designed a series of full-page ads that ran in our local paper encouraging two-child families. It's interesting how norms have changed: to younger readers this may sound like an effort to encourage families to have more children, but at the time it was about encouraging them to have fewer. And Mom made sure the ads were not subtle. The headlines read:

Have you considered the impact of the 3rd child on the environment?

Have you considered the impact of the 3rd child on our tax burden?

Have you considered the impact of the 3rd child on our freedoms?

Did I mention I was her third child? Nothing that thirty years of psychotherapy couldn't fix. I told you she was a character.

Mom went on to serve on Colorado's Certificate of Need panel and as trustee for Boulder Community Hospital. She gladly did battle with hospital administrators—and doctors—modeling a behavior that arguably was central to my own development. Boulder was a two-hospital town. I have vivid memories of dinnertime conversation when the "other" hospital wanted to get a CT scanner in the 1970s. Boulder Community already had one. Mom asked the question, "Do we really need two CT scanners in town?" She knew that was a recipe for twice as many CTs scans being performed—and twice as much money being spent.

In the 1980s, Mom got increasingly worried about medicine's tendency to do too much to people—particularly toward the end of life. She had long been a strong proponent of hospice and helping people avoid the indignities of a highly medicalized death. She also expressed more controversial beliefs: that patients should have some control on timing of their own death and that physician-assisted suicide should be legal. She became president of the Colorado Hemlock Society and got into a public debate with the archbishop of Denver over the issue. As my brother Pete is fond of saying, "That says it all."

In the 1990s some well-meaning Boulder physician wanted to help Mom live longer. When she was in her early seventies, he decided to start her on hormone replacement therapy—the administration of estrogen-containing compounds to women following menopause. That decision soon led to a phone call I'll never forget.

"Gilbert, it's like I'm having my period again!"

Yes, I was a medical professional. Yes, I had just joined the faculty of an Ivy League medical school. Yes, I had had more obstetrical and gynecological experience than average because of my time in the Indian Health Service. I just didn't want to have a conversation about vaginal spotting with my mother. I'm sorry.

But I did. I told her this was a side effect of hormone replacement therapy. She was not happy about that. She didn't want to have more laundry to do; she didn't want to use menstrual pads and tampons again.

"Do I really have to take this stuff?"

That was an interesting question. I understood where my mother's doctor was coming from. He had undoubtedly been reading what was the hot medical news at the time: hormone replacement therapy cuts the risk of cardiovascular disease in half.

Now cutting a risk in half is a big enough benefit to warrant further consideration—particularly when the disease is common, like heart disease. It could be restated as the inverse: *not* taking hormone replacement doubles your risk of heart disease. That's big enough to get my attention, particularly since heart disease is so common. But I also knew where my mother was coming from. And that's why it was an easy question to answer.

"No, Mom, you don't have to take that stuff."

That answer was easy. Why? Because there are a few basic principles fundamental to general questions about whether or not to pursue risk reduction interventions.

Patient autonomy: No one "has to do" anything. Discussions about biomedical ethics typically make my eyes glaze over, but for my profession, this is about as fundamental as it gets. I could see which way the wind was blowing on this phone call: she wanted to stop the medicine. Actually, I didn't think my mother could be made to do anything she didn't want to do anyway. But she was trained in an era when everyone—particularly nurses trained in wartime—was taught to follow the doctor's orders. She just needed permission from her doctor son to say no.

Baseline risk: How much an individual stands to benefit from a risk reduction effort is directly related to how high their current (or baseline) risk is. The higher the baseline risk, the higher the expected benefit. Patients with very high blood pressure, for example, stand to benefit a lot more from treatment than do patients with blood pressures slightly above average. I knew that Mom's risk of cardiovascular disease was, at worst, average. My best guess—given her family history, exercise behavior, and exercise tolerance—was that it was below average. Cutting a below average risk in half turns out to be a pretty small effect.

Certainty of the benefit: At the time, the information base about the value of hormone replacement therapy was solely based on observational data. In other words, studies that compared women who happened to take hormone replacement with those who did not found that women who took the drug had less heart disease. Observational data on preventive interventions are often subsequently found to be misleading (more on that in a minute). Bottom line: the benefit of hormone replacement was uncertain.

Certainty of the harm: Maybe you don't consider the side effect of vaginal spotting to be a harm, but Mom clearly did. And that harm wasn't a possibility, it was a certainty—it was actually occurring. The benefit might occur, but only in the future. The possibility of future benefit (and an uncertain one at that) versus a current harm?

For me, that's easy.

■ ■ ■

WHY DEVOTE SO MUCH TIME to a story about my mother? Because some version of it played out in approximately ten million American women. It was a massive effort to lower risk—an effort that ultimately proved to be one of the biggest medical errors on record.

EXPERIMENT TRUMPS OBSERVATION

Doll and Hill unleashed the power of observational data: the process of simply observing a population—some who are exposed, others who are not—as a way to deduce the effect of an exposure. They knew it was the only way to study exposures believed to be harmful to human health. Think about it: a committee to protect human subjects would never approve a human experiment in which half of the subjects were assigned to smoke cigarettes while the other half were not. And even if the study were approved, it would probably have difficulty recruiting subjects.

But the tools developed by Doll and Hill soon were applied to medical interventions hoped to be beneficial to human health—a situation in which a true experiment is not only ethically justifiable but imperative. The history of hormone replacement therapy serves as exhibit A.

During the 1980s and 1990s hundreds of studies were published linking hormone replacement to a lower risk of cardiovascular disease. Every journal seemed to have a favorable article to publish, every few months. That's what led Mom's doctor—and thousands of others—to start millions of women on hormone replacement. A review article in the *Journal of the American Medical Association* in 1991 summed up the evidence at the time:

> Most, but not all, studies of hormone replacement therapy in post-menopausal women show around a 50% reduction in risk of a coronary event in women using unopposed oral estrogen.

A few years later, the same journal published the findings of a computer model designed to estimate the effect of hormone replacement on the lifespan of a typical postmenopausal woman. The estimate was six months. That might not sound like much, but there are not many things doctors can do to make the average person live six months longer (other than getting cigarette smokers to quit, in which case life extension would be expressed in years). For the subgroup of women at very high risk for heart disease, the model suggested that hormone replacement might extend their life by as much as three years.

That's huge. It was almost too good to be true.

And it wasn't. The problem was that all the published articles were based on observational data. They all compared women who had been prescribed hormone replacement to those who had not. It turns out that women who were prescribed the drug differed in many ways from those who were not. They were wealthier (more likely to see a doctor to get the drug prescribed) and healthier (less likely to have other problems that would require their doctors to focus on more pressing issues than hormone replacement). They had better diets, exercised more, and were less likely to smoke. Of course, they had less heart disease. It had nothing to do with the drug.

We know that from true experiments, which are randomized trials. In these trials, women are divided into two groups—and the group to which they are assigned is determined purely by chance (that's what randomization means). One group is given hormone replacement; the other, a placebo.

Soon after the new millennium, the results of the randomized trials of hormone replacement were published. They made it clear that starting hormone replacement on women like my mother caused as many problems as it solved. Hormone replacement did reduce the risk of colon cancer and hip fracture, but it also increased the risk of stroke, breast cancer, and blood clots to the lung. And if anything, it increased the risk of heart disease.

Medicine is full of nuances, and thus I am compelled to add a couple of caveats here. First, it looks like the effect of hormone replacement depends on its timing. If it is started soon after menopause, its effects are more favorable. Second, the above-listed effects are relatively small (that is, 5 additional breast cancers per 1,000 women taking the drug over five years, meaning—when flipping the frame—no problem for

995). Infrequent harms experienced in the future can be trumped by symptomatic benefit experienced now. Who gets symptomatic benefit now? Those women who suffer severe menopausal symptoms (for example, hot flashes) and who feel better because of hormone replacement. It's a good drug for them.

But millions of women were like my mom. They had been started on hormone replacement years after menopause. They weren't being given the drug to make them feel better—they felt fine. They were being given the drug to prevent future problems.

And that turned out to be a huge mistake. Following publication of the randomized trials, millions of women came off hormone replacement. You could see the effect from space: the rate of breast cancer dropped nationwide.

There is a larger lesson in the hormone replacement saga: observational data can be very misleading for preventive interventions—interventions to reduce risk. The reason is that people who seek out preventive interventions (in our jargon, exhibit health-seeking behaviors) are very different from those who don't. In a word, they are healthier. So, of course, they do better. But the observation is misleading: while it's tempting to conclude they do better because of the preventive intervention, in fact they do better because they were destined to do better anyway (with or without the intervention).

It has been dubbed "prevention bias." And it's not just a problem with hormone replacement. Vitamin A, vitamin C, and vitamin E supplementation each appeared to produce big beneficial effects in observational data. But the effect disappeared in randomized trials. Why? Because people who take vitamins are healthier to begin with.

It's a problem for cancer screening. The people most interested in screening tend to be healthier than the general population—and have a lower risk for cancer. Two decades ago the federal government invited 150,000 men and women to participate in an experiment of screening for cancer in four organs: prostate, lung, colon, and ovary. The volunteers were less likely to smoke, more likely to exercise, had higher socioeconomic status, and fewer medical problems than members of the general population. Those are the kinds of people who seek preventive intervention. Of course, they are going to do better.

Had the study not been randomized, the investigators might have concluded that screening was the best thing since sliced bread. Regardless of which group they were randomly assigned to, the participants had substantially lower death rates than the general population—for all cancers (even those other than prostate, lung, colon, and ovary), for heart disease, and for injury. In other words, the volunteers were healthier than average. With randomization, the study showed that only one of the four screenings (for colon cancer) was beneficial. Without it, the study might have concluded that prostate cancer screening not only lowered the risk of death from prostate cancer but also deaths from leukemia, heart attack, and car accidents (although you would hope someone would raise the biological plausibility criterion here).

That's why you always want a randomized trial to make sure preventive interventions actually help people.

U-SHAPED CURVES

One of the contributions of chronic disease epidemiology has been the recognition that relationships between exposures and human health can get complex. Enter the U-shaped curve. When I enter the "U-shaped curve" on Google, I get something about happiness: high at the beginning of life, lowest in middle age, rises later in life. So we can infer that the horizontal axis is the time in life, the vertical axis is the amount of happiness, and the U shape translates to high at the extremes and low in the middle.

Let me be clear: I have no idea whether happiness is genuinely U-shaped. But I hope it is, because then I can only go up.

The "classic" U-shaped relationship in epidemiology is alcohol. The horizontal axis is the amount of alcohol consumption; the vertical axis is the rate of death. So now high is bad. A high level of alcohol consumption is definitely bad for you. But the lowest rate of death is not at the other extreme—abstainers. Instead the lowest part of the curve is somewhere in the middle—those who consume a moderate amount of alcohol, one to two drinks a day.

Excuse me while I grab a beer.

If you don't drink, I'm certainly not advocating that you start. The effect is not huge, and not certain enough, to advise that more people start drinking. Plus we know alcohol can create all sorts of problems. At the same time, however, people who drink in moderation have no reason to worry about it—and can even feel good about it.

But I didn't bring up U-shaped curves to discuss alcohol—or to rationalize my own behavior. I brought them up to discuss two biologic exposures: blood pressure and blood sugar. One of the first major American contributions to chronic disease epidemiology came from a small town twenty miles west of Boston—Framingham, Massachusetts. Oddly enough, my mother was born there but left too early to be part of this story. In 1948, the federal government recruited some five thousand residents between the ages of thirty and sixty-two to undergo extensive interviews and physical examinations. They then waited to find out who developed a heart attack or stroke. Much of what we now refer to as the risk factors for heart attack and stroke comes from the Framingham Heart Study.

In 1960 the first finding was published. Not surprisingly, the first risk factor identified was cigarette smoking. There were already reasons to stop smoking; this was just another nail in the coffin. A year later they published the second: high blood pressure. But just because high blood pressure had been identified as a risk factor for heart attack and stroke, doesn't mean that lowering blood pressure will help. Maybe blood pressure isn't the real culprit; maybe lowering blood pressure will harm people.

Remarkably, what happened next was exactly what should have happened. The government organized a randomized trial. The Department of Veterans Affairs (VA) conducted a cooperative study of men with really, really high blood pressure (diastolic blood pressure—the bottom number—over 115). Half got an active drug; half got a placebo. In less than two years the study was stopped. Why? Because the benefit of treating very high blood pressure was so big.

Treating very high blood pressure is one of the most important things doctors do. Very high blood pressure increases the risk of stroke, heart attacks, heart failure, and death in general. Lowering it has been shown to be beneficial in multiple randomized trials.

The effect is so dramatic that some were eager to extrapolate. If lowering very high blood pressure was good, it must be good to lower moderately high blood pressure, and if lowering moderately high blood pressure was good, it must be good to lower minimally high blood pressure. The mantra became: the lower the better.

Perhaps they thought about it like lead or cigarettes. We don't think there is some ideal, moderate exposure level for lead or cigarettes. We don't think there is a U-shaped curve; we think the relationship between these exposures and bad health outcomes is linear—or, more precisely, continually sloping upward—the higher the dose the worse the outcome.

But blood pressure is different. One of the first things medical students learn in acute care medicine is how bad it is to have very low blood pressure. Low blood pressure is hard on your vital organs—and it can cause people to fall. Both can cause death, particularly in the elderly. Of course the relationship is not linear; it's U-shaped.

A recent study delineated the left half of the U for patients with diabetes and heart disease. Having these two problems together unquestionably raises the risk of death, and lowering high blood pressure is the most important intervention doctors can do to lower that risk. The study found that it was good to lower blood pressure—to a point. Lower it beyond that point and the left half of the U-shaped curve appeared: death became more common. Where is that sweet spot—the trough of the U? We don't know exactly, but for patients with diabetes and heart disease it is probably a systolic blood pressure—the top number—between 120 and 140.

The medical profession has gotten very aggressive in treating blood pressure in diabetes. A recent VA study showed that overtreatment (too low) is now more common than undertreatment (too high). And it showed that the better a facility was at getting all diabetic patients below a target blood pressure, the more likely it was to be taking some patients too low. It's not rocket science; it's a U-shaped curve.

That's why the American Diabetes Association decided in 2012 to raise their recommended systolic blood pressure goal from under 130 to under 140. They were worried that the lower goal was producing very little benefit but was adding considerable harm. They wanted to make sure doctors didn't create risks by trying to lower them.

Those of us with elevated blood pressure without diabetes and heart disease are at lower risk for death and have less to gain from lowering blood pressure. Using the same rationale as the American Diabetes Association, I'd raise the systolic blood pressure goal for the rest of us from under 140 to under 150. At the end of 2013, amazingly, that became the recommendation for adults over age sixty.

Lowering blood pressure is not always a good thing. It depends on where you start (how high your blood pressure is)—and how much you lower it. The same is true for blood sugar.

Sugar, specifically glucose, is the fuel of all animal life. At low levels, the body is running on fumes—and vital organs get damaged, particularly the brain. At the same time, high levels are toxic to cells—and vital organs get damaged. It's another U-shaped curve.

With rare exception, the only people who have to worry about the left half of the U-shaped curve are those who take drugs to lower blood sugar—particularly those whose doctors are trying not simply to lower blood sugar but make it normal.

That was demonstrated dramatically in a randomized trial studying intensive versus standard therapy to lower blood sugar in patients with type 2 diabetes (that's the most common type of diabetes, the type that typically occurs in obese adults). For patients randomized to intensive therapy, the doctor's goal was to make their average blood sugar normal. The doctors were able to do that but at a human cost. The trial was stopped because the patients who had their glucose "normalized" also died more often. And it's not the only study that has shown that.

It is clearly not good to have very high blood sugar. It is clearly good to lower high blood sugar to normal through a combination of diet and exercise. But it clearly is not good to try to medicate diabetic patients until they have a normal blood sugar, because in doing so we will almost certainly cause some patients' blood sugar to get too low.

The relationship between exposures and human health can get complex. Sometimes lower is always better (lead and cigarettes), sometimes not (blood pressure and blood sugar). Because of the U-shaped curve, efforts to reduce small risks—like minimally elevated blood pressure and blood sugar—can produce big problems.

THE PRESENT TRUMPS THE FUTURE

I want to circle back to my favorite topic: me. There was another study of male doctors—the Physicians Health Study—published around the same time my mother was started on hormone replacement. It had found that regular aspirin lowers the risk of heart attacks. This wasn't an observational study, it was a true experiment: 22,000 physicians with no history of heart disease were randomized to receive either aspirin or placebo. So here the benefit of aspirin was as certain as it gets.

Just because the benefit was certain, however, doesn't mean everyone benefited. The study suggested that treating 1,000 men with aspirin for five years enabled about 10 to avoid a heart attack. The other 990 did not benefit.

That's not a huge effect: 10 benefited; 990 did not. But then again, taking aspirin is about as simple as it gets. So I, along with my colleagues, started putting a lot of patients on aspirin—as we will still do. I thought it was such a simple intervention I'd try it myself. After starting regular aspirin, however, I quickly experienced a harm: nosebleeds. I've always had nosebleeds. As a kid, Mom even took me to an ENT to get my nose cauterized (*that sure as hell didn't help*). I was started on vitamin K (*at least, that didn't hurt like hell*). My nosebleeds have always been more frequent in the winter, when heating dries out the house. Moving to the People's Republic of Vermont—and using the obligatory wood stove—didn't exactly improve the situation. Neither did aspirin, to say the least.

Aspirin inhibits platelet function, making it harder for the blood to clot. Good for heart attacks, bad for nosebleeds. After taking aspirin my nosebleeds became more frequent—and really, really hard to stop. I had to lie down and apply direct pressure for five, ten, even twenty minutes. I got nosebleeds at work; I got nosebleeds in my sleep. Big ones. Blood-stained ties, blood-stained dress shirts, blood-stained pillows, blood-stained bed sheets—what a bloody mess.

I'm sorry, am I sounding like my mother?

I didn't have to take this stuff. Sure there was a certain possibility of future benefit: about ten per one thousand over five years. But there was the certainty of a current harm. Maybe it seems ludicrous to trade off nosebleeds for heart attacks, but it was easy for me to do. Just as it is for my patients facing a similar situation—the few who develop frequent, severe nosebleeds can't wait to stop aspirin.

Sometimes trying to lower risk creates more problems than it solves.

As for my being overweight, don't worry about it. It's another U-shaped curve—plus we've defined "ideal" weight too narrowly. To be sure, obesity (BMI between 30 and 35)—and, particularly, severe obesity (BMI greater than 35)—is a problem to be dealt with. So too, however, is being underweight (BMI less than 18.5). But multiple studies have shown what is labeled overweight (BMI between 25 and 30) is actually associated with lower death rate than what is labeled normal weight (BMI between 18.5 and 25).

I'm not suggesting that you gain weight. Instead, I'm suggesting that we all be a little more cautious in asserting who is at high risk. Scaring people can have unpredictable effects. We sure as hell don't want people to start smoking as a way to lose weight.

PRESCRIPTION: FOCUS ON REDUCING BIG RISKS—FOR THOSE WHO ARE AVERAGE OR BELOW, LEAVE WELL ENOUGH ALONE

The world is not as dangerous a place as you may have been led to believe. To be sure, there are some exposures that are dangerous and should be avoided. Cigarette smoking is at the top of that list.

But many health risks you hear about are exaggerated. They reflect exposures with small effects—small enough that they may not even exist. If an exposure more than doubles your risk of something you care about—and it has been confirmed in multiple studies—you might want to pay attention. Otherwise ignore it. That will weed out much of the noise.

Risk reduction is challenging. Focusing on reducing big risks makes the most sense. Sometimes this simply involves avoiding things—like lead and cigarettes. Nothing has to be done to people; eliminating the exposure eliminates the risk. There is no harm from doing so (unless you want to posit an economic one for the lead and cigarette manufacturers).

But the minute something has to be done to you—an intervention like a drug, test, or procedure—you want to know whether the benefits are real and what harms exist. While you cannot expect evidence from a randomized trial for exposures believed to be harmful (committees for the protection of human subjects tend to frown on such studies), you should expect evidence from a randomized trial for preventive interventions believed to be beneficial. Remember: the fact that people who seek out the preventive intervention do better does not constitute evidence. That's the lesson from the hormone replacement saga. And for doctors the lesson is this: don't do the population until you do the trial.

For some exposures there's no such thing as too low. But exposures that follow a U-shaped curve—blood pressure and blood sugar—demand a more considered approach. Even for those at the highest risk, there is every reason to go slow and not let the perfect become the enemy of the good. Some have dubbed this minimally disruptive medicine—and even put it to music using the classic Eagles tune "Take It Easy." It's good advice.

It's hard for medical interventions to reduce average risks without creating new ones. While there is a lot of benefit to be had if you can reduce a high risk, there is little benefit in reducing an average risk. But the amount of harm from trying is roughly equivalent in the two situations. The truth is that interventions to reduce average risks can create as many problems as they solve.

Finally, this chapter has been focused on the future: you feel well now, but are concerned about what might happen. Symptoms change that equation—and in both directions. Women who suffer menopausal symptoms should not be scared about hormone replacement that allows them to feel better now. The reason is that the harms pale relative to the benefits. Conversely, those who suffer annoying side effects now from seemingly innocuous interventions, like aspirin, should not feel that by stopping them they have forgone some important benefit. Here the benefits pale relative to the harms. Symptoms in the present generally trump risks in the future.

It is prudent to accept low-level risks; we do it every day. A current TV ad sums it up nicely:

> There are man-eating sharks in every ocean, but we still swim. Every second somewhere in the world lightning strikes, but we still play in the rain. Poisonous snakes can be found in forty-nine of the fifty states, but we still go looking for adventure. A car can crash. A house can crumble. But we still drive and love coming home. Because I think deep down we know all the bad things that can happen in life, they can't stop us from making our lives good.

Sometimes Madison Avenue gets it right. It's not possible to eliminate all risk—nor is it desirable. And with medical care, trying creates risks of its own.

IT'S ALWAYS BETTER TO FIX THE PROBLEM

Disturbing truth: Trying to eliminate a problem can be more dangerous than managing one

WHEN FACED WITH A PROBLEM, my instinct is to want to fix it. And then move on to the next task. I don't think this is an attribute that is unique to doctors; I think it is fairly widespread.

When dealing with problems in your home, it's probably not a bad rule of thumb. If the roof is leaking, you should fix it—not leave buckets in the living room. If the kitchen sink drain is clogged, you should unclog it—not pour buckets of caustic chemicals like Drano on top of it. The same is true of your car. If the brake line is leaking, you should fix it—not just add more brake fluid. And if the windshield wiper motor dies, you should replace the motor—not rig up some half-baked solution like tying a rope to both wipers, passing it through the two triangular "vent" windows (*remember those?*), and then asking your high school buddy to pull the rope back and forth during a torrential rainstorm. I tried this once while crossing Wyoming on I-80 in my '65 Ford Fairlane . . . not smart.

On the other hand, fixing problems may not reliably be the best foreign policy strategy. We tried to fix the problem in Vietnam. We tried in

Iraq (admittedly there was considerable debate about what the problem was). I think we are learning as a country that you don't eliminate the problem of terrorism, you manage the problem.

OK. I'm no foreign policy expert. Or home and car repair expert, for that matter. But I know something about medical care—and I'm confident that not all medical problems should be fixed.

THE HEART OF THE MATTER

To provide some feel for the distinction between "fixing" and "managing" in medical care, I'm going to focus this chapter on a specialty that, to its credit, has devoted a lot of effort to investigating the question: cardiology. That means we need to start by talking about the heart.

The human heart is an impressive organ. It is the muscular pump that circulates our blood. Without any conscious effort, it just keeps pumping—as in 30 to 50 million contractions per year. I know, I'm guilty of pitching a "gee-whiz" number here—but gee whiz, it really is impressive when you think about it.

Muscles need a blood supply to work. They need oxygen, nutrition, and a way to get rid of waste products. The heart is no different. So while the vast majority of cardiac output goes elsewhere in the body, the heart also needs to pump blood to itself. This means that the heart has its own network of arteries—the coronary arteries. And, in the United States, this is the location where most heart problems occur; the most common type of heart disease is coronary artery disease.

The coronary arteries are not particularly big—the biggest is about a half a centimeter in diameter, or about one-fifth of an inch. So it doesn't take much to clog one and obstruct blood flow to the heart. That obstruction is coronary artery disease. A partial obstruction may cause the downstream muscle to receive too little oxygen, particularly with exertion—that's angina (chest pain). A sudden complete occlusion causes the downstream muscle to die—that's a heart attack.

Clearly, the ideal strategy would be to avoid the problem of coronary artery disease altogether. Avoiding coronary artery disease is the number 1 reason why we doctors feel so strongly about having people not smoke cigarettes (avoiding lung cancer is number 2). It's also why we care about diet and exercise. And it's why we aggressively give drugs to lower blood pressure and cholesterol (too aggressively from my standpoint, but that's a different story).

But no matter what we do, some people will eventually develop coronary artery disease. Then the question becomes: Should we manage the problem or try to fix it?

Managing the problem generally requires that medication be added to a healthy lifestyle. Once patients develop coronary artery obstruction, lowering cholesterol and blood pressure becomes particularly important. The first lowers the risk that the obstruction will progress; the second lowers the metabolic needs of the heart muscle—allowing it to do the job of pumping blood to the body, with less blood flowing to itself. Blood pressure is not the only determinant of metabolic needs; how fast the heart pumps matters as well. So we also give medicines that slow the heart rate.

Fixing the problem requires a mechanical intervention. That used to involve surgery, but increasingly it involves catheters. Catheters are long, thin, flexible tubes. To insert them into the heart, cardiologists start in the groin (or the wrist). That's why the tubes need to be long—as in over three feet long. Remember the coronary arteries are fairly small; that's why they need to be very thin. And it's not a straight shot going from an artery in the groin to an artery in the heart; that's why they need to be flexible.

If you have ever snaked a kitchen sink drain, you have some feel for what's going on. The catheters are sort of like drain augers—better known as sewer snakes—the instruments that plumbers and homeowners use to clear slow drains. Of course, a sewer snake is longer—ten to twenty-five feet—and a lot thicker. But the task is similar: a long flexible instrument needs to be guided through all sorts of twists and turns.

The cardiologists have an additional challenge: they are trying to get into one particular artery, one of many possibilities (while the plumbers only have one option: downstream toward the sewer). So the cardiol-ogists use X-rays in real time (fluoroscopy) to see where the catheter is and where it is going. With the help of a set of guide wires that have different dimensions and curvatures, they are able to redirect a catheter to get it to go where they want it to go. Once the catheter tip arrives at the obstruction, they inflate a balloon to relieve the obstruction. Fre-quently, they then insert a second catheter with a stent—not unlike a small metal spring—to keep the artery open.

Balloon angioplasty is a pretty amazing procedure. I feel fortunate to have cardiologist friends who have invited me to watch it. (Although, given my sewer snake analogy, that sentence probably should be edited to "have had cardiologist friends.") However, things can go wrong.

The last time I faced a clogged kitchen sink full of water, I made the mistake of trying to snake through an ill-fitting trap. It popped off and the water promptly drained all over the floor.

Similarly, balloon angioplasty can damage the blood vessels. Some-times this causes bleeding, sometimes it causes a stroke, sometimes it causes a heart attack. Sometimes patients have to undergo emergency surgery to repair a problem. Rarely someone dies. It's all on the con-sent form.

But if I were having a heart attack, I'd sign it ASAP. I'd want to fix the problem.

Why do I say this? Because there are high quality data showing that fixing the problem of a heart attack is a better strategy than managing it. By high quality data, I mean data from a true experiment: a random-ized trial. In these trials, patients having heart attacks are divided into two groups—and the group to which they are assigned is determined purely by chance. In one group the heart attack is managed medically (using a "clot busting" drug); in the other group a cardiologist tries to fix the problem with balloon angioplasty.

Randomized trials are by far the best way to determine what works in medicine. They are the most reliable way to construct two groups that are similar in every way except one—how they were treated. Thus any differences observed at the end of the study must be the *result* of how they were treated.

To understand why randomization is so important, it is useful to consider the alternative: compare patients who happen to have their heart attack medically managed with those who happen to have their heart attack fixed. The problem is that these groups can differ in many important ways other than how they are treated. The medically managed group could be those patients who are too old or too sick to undergo angioplasty. These patients are bound to do poorly. So even if angioplasty did not help anyone, it would appear to work better than medical management. So while this kind of comparison is convenient, it is not a reliable way to learn what works.

There have been over twenty randomized trials comparing balloon angioplasty versus medical management for heart attack. That's a tribute to the field—and to the patients who agreed to participate in the research. A meta-analysis—a summary analysis combining all the data as if it were a single large trial—was published in the journal *Lancet*. It found that angioplasty patients were less likely to have a second heart attack in the month following their first: 3 percent in the angioplasty group versus 7 percent in the medical management group. Angioplasty patients were also less likely to die in the month following their heart attack: 7 percent versus 9 percent.

At first blush, 7 percent versus 9 percent might not sound like a huge effect—particularly after I said in the last chapter that I'd filter out anything that didn't at least double (or halve) my risk. But that was when I was the average-risk patient—when I was well, when most bad health events are thankfully rare: as in, occur to less than 1 percent in the next decade. And I also mentioned that baseline risks matter.

Now I'm having a heart attack. My baseline risk has just skyrocketed: now we're talking about a 7 percent versus 9 percent risk of dying *in the next thirty days*. Unless death has become a desirable outcome for me—and at some point it likely will—I'll take the 7 percent, thanks.

That's why, if I were having a heart attack, I'd want them to run the snake up my groin. Fix the problem.

THE PARTIAL PROBLEM

Angina patients are much more common than heart attack patients. In other words, partial obstruction of the coronary arteries is much more common than complete obstruction. Should we manage the problem of angina or try to fix it?

Since most balloon angioplasties in the United States are done for angina—not heart attacks—you can imagine this would be a fairly threatening question for cardiologists. In fact, it's bigger than that. Ask any hospital administrator what their big revenue generators are. They'll tell you the radiology department, the outpatient surgery center, the endoscopy suites, and the rooms where cardiologists guide these catheters—the cath lab.

Given the financial interests at stake, it took courage to even ask the question. The randomized trial that addressed it was titled "Clinical Outcomes Utilizing Revascularization and Aggressive Drug Evaluation." Trialists are getting very clever choosing titles that result in catchy, easy-to-remember acronyms—this one spells COURAGE. (My persnickety editor pointed out that it actually spells COURADE, leading me to have to figure out that the trialists stole the G from the second letter of "Aggressive," dropped the D in "Drugs," and are expending too much effort in creating acronyms.)

COURAGE randomized patients who had stable angina—that means chest pain that occurs with exertion and goes away at rest—and at least one partial obstruction of a coronary artery, meaning that the artery had been narrowed by at least 70 percent.

The patients who had their obstruction "fixed" with balloon angioplasty were no less likely to die or have a heart attack than patients who had their obstruction "managed" with medical therapy, the cholesterol- and blood pressure–lowering medications mentioned before. If there was any benefit to fixing the problem it was in terms of quality of life: both groups of patients felt markedly better following therapy, but the angioplasty patients got better quicker. Two to three years later, the two groups felt the same. Remember: the effort to fix the problem comes with the upfront risk of heart attack, stroke, and (rarely) death.

The accompanying editorial in the *New England Journal of Medicine* summed it up this way:

> For every 1000 patients treated with a PCI-first strategy [balloon angioplasty], approximately 2 would die, 28 would have a periprocedural myocardial infarction [a heart attack caused by the procedure], 60 to 90 would have an incremental, transient gain in health status, and 800 or more would see neither harm nor benefit.

If I developed stable angina, I'd start with medical management. I'd pass on being snaked.

Time for another nuance paragraph. Notice I used the word *start*. Medical management often works very well in controlling symptoms, but not always. If I still had bothersome symptoms on medical therapy, I'd certainly consider balloon angioplasty. That's exactly what happened to the medical therapy group in COURAGE: about one-third went on to have an angioplasty in the next five years. That's sensible—if Plan A doesn't work, move on to Plan B. That's step-wise medical care. Don't miss the fact that this strategy allows two-thirds to avoid the procedure.

COURAGE was a "game changer" in cardiology. It made it clear that angioplasty did not help avoid death or heart attacks in angina patients. The only reason to do it was for symptoms—to help people feel better. That was big news. You could see the effect from space: trends in nationwide data that my Dartmouth colleagues and I regularly monitor. Following the publication of COURAGE, the number of balloon angioplasties dropped by about one-quarter—more than 200,000 fewer procedures per year.

But the coronary artery disease game has not totally changed. Doctors still get a lot of pressure to just fix the problem. Dr. Walton-Shirley, a cardiologist in private practice in Glasgow, Kentucky, described the tension for Medscape, a web resource for health professionals:

It's difficult to practice COURAGE trial cardiology. Case in point: I recently evaluated a very nice older gentleman who was accompanied by his daughter for his first office visit. Just by age and risk factors alone, it's a sure bet that if I cathed him, he'd have a veritable playground of coronary disease, enough fodder to give any plumber a nice fat return on their work.

That's good; a cardiologist uses the plumbing analogy. I feel on more solid ground.

After Dr. Walton-Shirley performed a careful evaluation—which included imaging the heart under stress—she decided to manage the problem with medications. She was pleased with the result:

> On our last interview, he was having no symptoms. His blood pressure was now 120/70s. I explained the probability of coronary disease and even mentioned a cath if he had progressive symptoms. He expressed no interest in it. He left my office with a plan for a short follow-up in eight weeks. I felt we had accomplished much. With a normal BP, no symptoms, and an approximately 40% lower risk of MI (heart attack) and cardiac death on his new meds, what more could one ask?

You could ask that the problem be fixed. Apparently that is what the patient's daughter wanted. So she sought a second opinion and found someone who would do an angioplasty. Dr. Walton-Shirley expressed her frustration—and her concern for her patient:

> He risked stroke and other complications to make his daughter feel like she had done something for her dad. . . . Everyone who was involved with this patient to this very moment is telling and retelling the story, "Oh my gosh, If I hadn't taken him to this other doctor, he would have been a ticking time bomb!" Makes for a good story, but the thing that should have been done had been done already. His new medication regimen consisting of a beta blocker and amlodipine is cheap,

effective, but not glamorous enough for the many who never heard of the COURAGE trial, never bothered to read the COURAGE trial, or who are not brave enough to practice COURAGE trial medicine. Furthermore, you'd never convince anyone in his party, now that the surgery is over, that the patient could likely have coexisted peacefully with those "terrible" blockages and likely could have gone on for years or maybe even a lifetime without an event.

There is no more of a true believer than a patient who has undergone a major therapeutic intervention—be it for heart disease, back pain, or cancer. These patients have been through a big deal. So if they do well afterward, of course, they want to attribute doing well to their decision to undergo the treatment.

Patient stories of "success" are very powerful, but they can also be very misleading. Few want to raise the alternative possibility: the patient didn't need the intervention in the first place—they were going to be fine without intervention, perhaps they would be even better. No one, particularly doctors, has any interest in raising the possibility that they went through all that for nothing.

THE NO-PROBLEM PROBLEM

Ironically, as interventions become more commonplace, more people have heard a success story and more people are primed to think the intervention is right for them. Add that to the widely held assumption that it's always better to fix problems and you get too much medical care.

Maybe that's why President George W. Bush had a balloon angioplasty in 2013. He didn't even have a problem. He was sixty-seven years old at the time and was in remarkable shape: he cleared brush on the ranch, he was an avid bike rider, and he had no symptoms.

This is in sharp contrast to his vice president. Mr. Cheney had boatloads of symptoms. He had multiple bouts of angina and multiple heart attacks—his first was at age thirty-seven. That is extremely young. And he had multiple angioplasties and cardiac bypass surgery. He undoubtedly needed them.

Of course, I have no direct knowledge of either case. All I know is what appears in the press. From the press reports it looked like the former president went in for a routine physical, which included a cardiac stress test (which is certainly not routine in an asymptomatic patient). It showed some abnormality—as it would in many sixty-seven-year-olds—and Mr. Bush was off to have his coronary artery anatomy detailed. He was off to the cath lab. The catheterization identified a partial obstruction—as I expect it might in me—and a balloon was inflated.

I'm afraid that sequence of events is wholly unremarkable in the wild west of American medicine. What is remarkable is that some doctors were willing to say exactly what they thought about it. Dr. Richard Besser, the chief medical correspondent for ABC News and former director of the Centers for Disease Control (CDC), questioned the procedure:

> In people who are not having symptoms, the American Heart Association says you should not do a stress test since the value of opening that artery is to relieve the symptoms.

Dr. Vinay Prasad and Dr. Adam Cifu, from the National Cancer Institute and University of Chicago, respectively, wrote an op-ed for the *Washington Post* questioning the procedure:

> It is worth noting that at least two large randomized trials show that stenting these sorts of lesions does not improve survival. Because Mr. Bush had no symptoms, it is impossible that he felt better after these procedures.
>
> Instead, George W. Bush will have to take two blood thinners, aspirin and Plavix, for at least a month and probably a year. While he takes these medications, he will have a higher risk of bleeding complications with no real benefit.

But what do these guys know? They're not cardiologists (nor am I). Amazingly, however, cardiologists were asking questions too. Dr. Paul Chan, from the Mid America Heart Institute, questioned the procedure:

> The reality is that we don't know if we can change the trajectory of disease in people who don't have symptoms, are doing fine and are physically active. . . . There's no evidence treatment will help them live longer, feel better, or have fewer heart attacks.

And Dr. Steven Nissen, the head of cardiology at the Cleveland Clinic, did not hesitate to say what he really thought:

> This is really American medicine at its worst. It's one of the reasons we spend so much on health care and we don't get a lot for it. In this circumstance, the stent doesn't prolong life, it doesn't prevent heart attacks and it's hard to make a patient who has no symptoms feel better.

Hard to make a patient who has no symptoms feel better. There's nothing I can add to that.

THE ELECTRICAL PROBLEM

Since I wrote about a Republican, I have to write about a Democrat. It's part of the Federal Communication Commission's equal time requirement. So let's move from President Bush to Vice President Biden.

I really like Joe. He relishes being seen as an average Joe—riding Amtrak to work, buying coffee at Dunkin Donuts, shopping at Costco. And he's so refreshingly frank. I loved the time he whispered (not quietly enough) in President Obama's ear, "This is a big fucking deal," following the passage of the Affordable Patient Care Act. To be sure, as the first major piece of health-care legislation since Medicare/Medicaid, it was.

I also like refreshingly frank doctors. I'll never forget the time I overheard two colleagues talking and one said to the other, "It was a textbook case of *iatrogenesis fulminans.*"

Iatrogenesis fulminans. I'd never heard the term before, but I knew what it meant—and I knew I wanted to hear more.

You won't find the term in a medical dictionary. *Iatrogenesis* means "originating from a physician" and could conceivably include both beneficial and harmful effects. But in common usage, *iatrogenesis* refers to harm emanating from medical care. *Fulminans* comes from the Latin root *fulmen* meaning lightning or thunderbolt. In medical contexts I think of it as meaning "full on." *Acne fulminans* is not a subtle case of acne; it's a full-on case of acne—an extreme case.

Iatrogenesis fulminans is medical slang that reflects the gallows humor of physicians. It's when something we do goes terribly wrong—typically in a situation where we didn't *have* to do something, but chose to. These two doctors were talking about a cardiologist's effort to fix—not a plumbing problem, but an electrical one.

The heart is a sophisticated pump. It is split into two halves: the left half pumps oxygenated blood (coming from the lungs) to the rest of the body, the right half pumps deoxygenated blood (coming from the body) to the lungs. And each half has two chambers: the smaller atrium on top and the larger ventricle below. For the heart to work well, these chambers need to pump sequentially. And to respond to the increased demands of exertion, the heart will increase its rate of pumping (which is a good thing or I'd never have the oomph required to climb a hill).

Clearly, to make this variable speed, four-chamber, sequential pump work—it is going to take a serious electrical system. That's right: your heart is wired.

So while most heart problems involve the pump muscle not getting enough blood to work well (read: heart attack or angina), sometimes the problem involves the electrical system. The pump is fine, but its rhythm is wrong—because the electrical system is telling the heart to pump too fast, too slow, or erratically. These rhythm problems are lumped together under the general heading of cardiac arrhythmias.

The most feared arrhythmias emanate from the ventricles. Because the ventricles are the large chambers of the heart—the ones that do the heavy lifting—ventricular arrhythmias can be lethal. The most common cardiac arrhythmia, however, emanates from the atria; it may, or may not, cause symptoms.

It's called atrial fibrillation—meaning the two top chambers are producing rapid, irregular, and unsynchronized electrical activity. That has two consequences. First, when there is a lot of erratic electrical activity in the atria, some of it will pass through a relay station—called the AV node—on to the ventricles. That makes the heart beat irregularly—and because there is no pattern to the irregularity, we say the rhythm is irregularly irregular (I've always loved that phrase). And if too much electrical activity passes to the ventricles, that can cause the heart to beat too fast. Fast, erratic heart rates can cause symptoms: palpitations, light-headedness, and shortness of breath.

Second, the unsynchronized electrical activity means that the atria don't contract; they quiver (which is like "shiver," only not due to cold). Because the bottom two chambers—the ventricles—are the powerful part of the pump, this has a relatively small effect on overall pump function. In other words, the loss of atrial contraction doesn't typically cause symptoms. But it does mean that blood doesn't move much in the chamber. Blood that sits in one place has a tendency to clot. And blood clots in the heart can break loose and travel up to the brain, leading to the most feared consequence of atrial fibrillation—a stroke.

Should we manage the problem of atrial fibrillation or try to fix it?

Managing the problem involves a two-prong strategy. The first is rate control—preventing the ventricles from beating too fast (typically using beta-blockers, a class of medication that has been around for years). The second is anticoagulation—colloquially referred to as "thinning the blood." This lowers the risk of blood clotting in the sluggish atria and thus lowers the risk of stroke. Anticoagulation carries its own risk, however: serious bleeding.

Fixing the problem—stopping the atria from fibrillating and getting back to a normal heart rhythm—would seem preferable. Patients would avoid the risk of anticoagulation. The conventional fix to the problem involves a class of drugs called *antiarrhythmics.*

I am scared of prescribing antiarrhythmic drugs (note: I'm not including beta-blockers or calcium channel blockers here). I never start a patient on one; I let the cardiologists do that. I don't even like refilling prescriptions for antiarrhythmics. I bet a lot of primary care practitioners feel that way.

The reason is this: antiarrhythmics are a mixed bag. They are not well tolerated by patients and they have an unfortunate side effect: they can cause arrhythmias (in another classic phrase from our jargon, antiarrhythmics can be proarrhythmic). Lethal arrhythmias. Wiki-ing the term "antiarrhythmic agent," I see this: According to at least one source, cardiac anti-arrhythmia drugs have "cost more American lives than the Vietnam War." One of the cardiologists who kindly reviewed this chapter commented at this juncture, "Are you sure you want to cite *Wikipedia?*" . . . after writing, "I don't doubt it."

No one knows what the true number is, but antiarrhythmic drugs are definitely more dangerous than most medications. They definitely do kill people.

But then again so do anticoagulation drugs. In principle, at least, there is a good rationale for making the heart rhythm normal—so that the heart can pump as designed and avoid the risks of anticoagulation.

A pair of randomized trials—one from the United States, the other from Europe—compared the fix versus manage strategy for the typical patient with atrial fibrillation. They were published simultaneously in the *New England Journal of Medicine.*

Fixing the problem didn't look so good. The trial that measured mortality showed that there were more deaths in the fix-it group. This could be due to chance, but I doubt it (for the statisticians among you, the p value was 0.08; for the rest of you, this means that the probability that this result was due to chance was only 8 percent). The other trial showed that there were more bad events overall in the fix-it group (a combination of death from heart disease plus episodes of heart failure, strokes, major bleeding, and dangerous arrhythmias). That could be due to chance, but I doubt it (again, for the statisticians, the p value was 0.11).

What was most surprising was that the effort to fix the problem offered no advantage in terms of the primary goal of atrial fibrillation treatment: to reduce the amount of stroke. That's because a lot of patients in the fix-it group never got fixed (they remained in atrial fibrillation) or got fixed only transiently (they go back and forth between a normal rhythm and atrial fibrillation). So there's another reason antiarrhythmics are a mixed bag—they don't reliably work.

If I develop atrial fibrillation, I want it managed.

But some patients still want to try to fix the problem—to really fix it, not with a drug but with a procedure. And there are some cardiologists who are happy to try. That's where the textbook case of *iatrogenesis fulminans* comes in.

Larry had atrial fibrillation. Although he could be managed with rate control drugs and anticoagulation, he was bothered by the palpitations: the sensation of his heart pounding. He searched the web for new treatments and came across advertisements like this:

We can treat your atrial fibrillation at the Electrophysiology Lab at Doctors Hospital at White Rock Lake.

The Stanford Arrhythmia Service is here to return the rhythm to your everyday life.

Medstar Heart Institute—Restoring the Rhythm of Life.

Larry wanted the problem fixed.

The new strategy to fix atrial fibrillation is called catheter ablation. Ablation means destruction. In this case, doctors are trying to destroy the electrical circuits from which atrial fibrillation originates—typically near where the pulmonary veins open into the left atrium. Destruction sounds problematic enough, but so too is just getting to the work site.

Even with a long, thin, flexible catheter, it's not easy to get to the opening of the pulmonary veins. If you started in an artery (the approach for balloon angioplasty), you would have to go through the aortic valve, through the left ventricle, and finally through the mitral valve. The whole effort is in the wrong direction: against the flow of blood.

So the approach is to start in a vein. Now the problem is that you are approaching the wrong side of the heart. You can get to the right atrium easily, but then you need to puncture the wall of the heart to get into the left atrium. That's called transseptal catheterization. Then you are destroying something you can't see directly, only on an X-ray screen.

Larry went to a heart hospital in Texas to have the ablation. The procedure seemed to go well. Like most ablation patients, he continued anticoagulation therapy to reduce the risk of stroke. A few weeks later he was vomiting up blood. Turns out that the esophagus—the swallowing tube—sits right behind the opening of the pulmonary veins. Larry had developed an atrio-esophageal fistula: blood was leaking from the left atrium of his heart into his esophagus. Apparently, there was a little too much destruction.

That's not good. And it's not easy to fix that problem. It requires major chest surgery—as in six to eight hours of surgery. Surgery that can lead to death simply from uncontrolled bleeding: exsanguination. Luckily Larry survived, but he will never be the same.

That's *iatrogenesis fulminans.*

Ironically, the same week I learned about Larry from my two colleagues, I also learned about Pam from her husband. She had atrial fibrillation. She wanted it fixed. She went to Johns Hopkins. She had her pulmonary veins ablated. She also required major chest surgery: not to repair an atrio-esophageal fistula, but to repair the mitral valve. After the wall of the heart was punctured, the catheter didn't stay in the left atrium—it slipped through the mitral valve (moving with the flow of blood) and into the left ventricle. When the cardiologist tried to pull the catheter back, it got caught on the web of muscles that support the valve. Pulling the catheter out tore up the structures that support the valve. When that happens, blood pumps in the wrong direction.

Sudden and severe damage to the mitral valve is not compatible with life; it must be repaired—involving another major chest surgery. Luckily Pam survived, but she will never be the same.

That's *iatrogenesis fulminans.*

I don't enjoy writing these stories. They lack context. In many ways they are no better than the patient success stories I was complaining about a few pages ago. You should understand that the only doctor that never has a role in causing harm is the doctor who no longer sees patients. But I also recognize that the public needs some feel for what can go wrong in order to have a better understanding for why aggressive intervention is generally not the first choice—why it is not always better to try to fix the problem.

Here is the larger context. There is a small, select group of patients who might want to consider the ablation procedure. They are relatively young, have no other medical problems, and are in a normal heart rhythm most of the time. Their problem is that they occasionally flip into atrial fibrillation without warning, develop a very rapid heart rate, and become very light-headed. Using drugs to prevent the heart from racing during these rare episodes may cause it to beat too slowly most of the time—and also make these patients light-headed. Ablation can stop their hearts from flipping into atrial fibrillation, but the procedure typically needs to be done more than once. Even for these patients, there are real reasons to proceed with caution.

In my book, pulmonary artery ablation qualifies as a dangerous procedure—a strategy of last resort. Atrio-esophageal fistula is not common, but there are multiple reports of it in the medical literature. Damage to the mitral valve is not common, but there are multiple reports of it in the medical literature. More common complications include cardiac tamponade (when the heart can no longer pump well because the sack around it is full of blood) and pulmonary vein stenosis (when the vaporization causes the vein to scar, thus obstructing blood flow, raising blood pressure in the lung, and impeding lung function).

You might reasonably ask: How often do these complications happen? The fact that I can't reliably answer that question is—from my standpoint—the single best argument for a single-payer health-care system. If every procedure was tracked by a single payer, it would be possible to know what's actually happening to people who undergo the procedure—at least in terms of how often they need subsequent procedures to fix something that went wrong with the first.

Instead we are left with data from single institutions. These err in only one direction: they are underestimates. There are numerous explanations for this. Clinicians tend to underreport, not overreport, complications. Thus investigators tend to miss complications; but they don't fabricate them. The studies typically have short follow-up, while some complications take years to occur. Finally, the institutions that tend to do analyses of complications tend to be high-volume prestigious academic medical centers, which tend to be those with low complication rates.

I found two single institution reports of complications following catheter ablation for atrial fibrillation: one from Hopkins, the other from Harvard (see what I mean?). Both report only major complications: *those that were life-threatening, resulted in permanent harm, required intervention, or significantly prolonged hospitalization.* Both reported that major complication occurred in about 5 percent of procedures. And both reported that 1 percent of patients had a stroke following the procedure.

Stroke? Wasn't that what we were trying to prevent? That's right, the procedure itself causes stroke. It's another complication. And it gets worse: the expert consensus panel that was convened to make recommendations for catheter ablation for atrial fibrillation recommends continuing anticoagulation after the procedure. These are the doctors who do the procedure, who believe in the procedure. Why do they do that? Because they know the procedure does not reliably fix the problem.

If we are not solving the feared consequence of atrial fibrillation, if we still need to continue anticoagulation, what are we doing putting a snake through the wall of the heart and destroying the opening of major veins next to the esophagus? All for what is fundamentally a nonlethal arrhythmia.

And what are we doing advertising the procedure in the subway? Here's the promotion currently posted in Washington, DC's Metro: *A Fib felt like a tsunami crashing in my chest.*

We sure as hell better be making people feel a *whole* lot better. But even that's not clear. Note: there are two prerequisites to feeling a whole lot better: first, you need to start off feeling like you have a tsunami (i.e., have severe symptoms), and second, the procedure needs to reliably solve the problem without causing another tsunami.

Promoting this fix to this problem sure seems like a recipe for *iatrogenesis fulminans.* And don't make the mistake of thinking the concern is only relevant to cardiology.

THE LIMITATIONS OF RESEARCH

There are two broad categories of medical research: observational research and true experiments. For observational research, think Doll and Hill: observe a population—some who are exposed, some who are not—and see what happens to each group. There is no attempt to direct who is in which group. For true experiments, think randomized trial: randomly allocate individuals to one strategy versus another and see what happens to each group. Here patients are directed to one group or another—simply by the play of chance.

This chapter was informed by randomized trials. Credit the cardiologists who design and manage them—as well as the patients who participate in them.

In the previous chapter, I argued that you always want a randomized trial to make sure preventive interventions actually help people. In this chapter, I'll broaden the argument: randomized trials are the best source of information about the true effect of any medical intervention. Truth is, I am a card-carrying member of a movement in medicine to embrace evidence-based medicine.

Some of my colleagues enjoy mocking this movement—they call us "EBMers"—because our knee-jerk response to any medical question is either to quote a randomized trial or suggest that one needs to be done. That response is too easy to make—and it's too easy to make fun of.

The *British Medical Journal* ran a wonderful parody of evidence-based medicine in their 2003 Christmas issue—which always features spoofs. The article was titled "Parachute Use to Prevent Death and Major Trauma Related to Gravitational Challenge: Systematic Review of Randomized Controlled Trials." It gravely reported, "We were unable to identify any randomized controlled trials of parachute intervention" and then went on to conclude:

> As with many interventions intended to prevent ill health, the effectiveness of parachutes has not been subjected to rigorous evaluation by using randomized controlled trials. Advocates of evidence based medicine have criticized the adoption of interventions evaluated by using only observational data. We think that everyone might benefit if the most radical protagonists of evidence based medicine organized and participated in a double blind, randomized, placebo controlled, crossover trial of the parachute.

Placebo controlled—that would be like a backpack containing a nonfunctional parachute. And the recommendation of the crossover trial is a nice touch. It means a subject randomized to one group will, after a period of observation, cross over to join the other group. Very effective: no matter what the randomization, doctors like me would ultimately find themselves in the control group—and get to jump out of a plane without a parachute.

The evidence-based medicine critics have a point: randomized trials are not always possible. We can't randomize people to receive what we believe might be a harmful exposure, like jumping out of a plane without a parachute or taking up the habit of cigarette smoking. And the more sophisticated critics would be quick to point out three other limitations to randomized trials.

First, they may focus on the wrong comparison. There have been a number of randomized trials of catheter ablation in atrial fibrillation. The comparison group typically consists of patients taking antiarrhythmic drugs. Why would I be interested in that comparison? We already know that antiarrhythmic drugs don't work that well in atrial fibrillation—and that they have loads of side effects (including death). What I want to know is how ablation compares to the standard treatment of rate control and anticoagulation.

Second, they may focus on the wrong outcome. The typical outcome measure for randomized trials of catheter ablation in atrial fibrillation is whether patients still have the arrhythmia or not—as determined by an electrocardiogram (EKG) tracing of the electrical activity of the heart. But patients don't care about what their EKG looks like, they care about how they feel. And they care about their chance of having a stroke, their chance of having a complication—and their chance of death. I'm happy to report there is an ongoing Canadian trial of catheter ablation versus rate control that is focused on outcomes that matter: mortality, hospitalization, and quality of life. It will include about a thousand patients and is expected to be completed in 2016.

Third, they may focus on the wrong patients. One of the pharmaceutical industry's favorite strategies is to study the effect of a drug on the few patients who have severe disease, find some benefit, and then hope that doctors extrapolate the benefit to the many patients with less severe forms of the disease. It's a clever strategy: it's like testing parachutes on the few people who jump out of airplanes and then selling them as protection against falls to the many people who walk downstairs. Severely ill patients always stand to benefit more from intervention than those who are less severely ill (it's all about baseline risk, remember?). Yet the harms of intervention are roughly equivalent in the two groups. So the net effect of intervention regularly looks better in the severely ill. To be sure, the problem can work in the reverse direction: if a trial focuses on patients who are only moderately ill, and then finds no benefit, it may have missed an important effect among the severely ill.

Finally, the results of randomized trials reflect the typical patient that is enrolled in the study. In other words, they show the average effect of intervention. Some individuals may do much better; others may do much worse. But when we are trying to infer the effect of a new treatment—giving a drug, performing a procedure—it is highly desirable to have data from a randomized trial. Randomized trials are far from perfect, but they are the best source of information we have.

PRESCRIPTION: ASK ABOUT OPTIONS AND START SLOW

There are always options. And while there are a few medical emergencies in which interventions must be done quickly, for the vast majority of medical care you have time to consider them. But you can't consider options unless you ask what they are.

Most people assume that a medical intervention directed to fix a problem will be more beneficial than one that simply manages it. As you've seen in this chapter, this assumption may or may not be true. However, a lot of medicine is even murkier. There often won't even be a clear answer: there will be advantages and disadvantages to each option, studies will disagree about which option is better, or there will be no studies at all.

Against this backdrop it is important to remember that while all medical interventions have harms, some are more harmful than others. In general, an intervention that attempts to fix a problem will be associated with a higher risk for something bad happening. Fixing things is a bit of a gamble. There's a chance that it makes you a whole lot better, but there's also a chance it makes you a whole lot worse.

That's why, in general, my advice is a stepwise approach: start slow. Try the more conservative options first. You can always ratchet it up later.

When you do consider fixing something—that is, having a major elective procedure—take the time to get more than one opinion about it. Think of it like buying a car or a house. Act as if it were a major purchase. It is—even if someone else is paying for it. Get an opinion from an independent source: a doctor who doesn't perform the procedure. And ask whether there are any relevant randomized trials.

It's also good to be clear about exactly what you are trying to fix— what the goal is. In my simple view of the world, there are only two reasons to subject patients to intervention: (1) to help them live longer and (2) to help them feel better. So if you feel good now, you have every reason to demand high-quality evidence from a randomized trial that fixing your "problem" will help you live longer.

Ask about options, take the time—and, when in doubt, start slow.

ASSUMPTION #3

SOONER IS ALWAYS BETTER

*Disturbing truth: Early diagnosis can
needlessly turn people into patients*

THIS CHAPTER MAY CHALLENGE your assumptions about screening—specifically, cancer screening.

Were my daughter here (and not in the wilds of northeast Australia), she would undoubtedly have something like this to say: "*Dad, don't you think it's time for you to find something new to write about? You keep saying the same things over and over and over . . .*"

I know I sound like a broken record on this issue. (I also know that my daughter has no clue what a broken record is . . . despite the fact that I have a number of the aforementioned vinyl artifacts in my study.) For a quarter century, cancer screening has been the central thrust of my research and my writing for the public. Nevertheless, I know—from reading newspapers, watching television, seeing bills passed in Congress, and observing cancer advocacy campaigns—that a lot of misconceptions persist. If you have read either of my prior books, you undoubtedly know where I'm going—so feel free to move on.

If you haven't, your intuition might be that cancer screening is a "no-brainer." You might think that screening only works in one direction: it can only make things better. You might think screening can only lower your risk of getting cancer. You might think that all the "cancer survivors" in the news (and, perhaps, in your neighborhood)—those individuals whose cancers were found early by screening and who are now doing well—provide powerful evidence that screening helps save lives.

In this chapter, I'm going to ask you to think again.

Intuition is a powerful thing. It can be very useful; it can be very misleading. In this case, it's the latter—because screening is counterintuitive. It turns out that screening works in two directions: it has both benefits and harms. And unfortunately, the harms are much more certain than the benefits. It turns out that screening is the fastest way to get cancer. Furthermore, it turns out that the survivors whose cancers were caught by screening are less likely to be evidence of its benefit—and more likely to be evidence of its harms.

Maybe you think I'm crazy. Or maybe the way we think about cancer is crazy. Maybe we need to develop a new conceptual model of the disease. Oddly enough, that is exactly what's happening.

SCREENING: ALWAYS A GOOD IDEA

Not infrequently, health reporters contact me. Typically, they are contacting me about screening: either about my research, the research of others, a new recommendation—whatever puts screening in the news. I view answering them as part of my job.

Yeah, it takes time away from other things. And that time generally involves not just the time talking with the reporter, but also the time to figure out exactly what I should say. This is particularly true when the story is not about my research—when figuring out what to say involves a little research in itself (such as reviewing the work of other investigators and what else is known about the topic).

I say it's part of my job for two reasons. First, I believe academic physicians have some obligation to communicate what we are learning to the general public—both because it is the right thing to do and because many of us are ultimately supported by public funds (either via federal grants, through Medicare payments for teaching hospitals or, as was my case for twenty-seven years, because we are federal employees).

But there is another reason it's part of my job: it is in my interest. I'm not talking about financial interest here—being able to say that is one reason I didn't want to make money from selling books—I'm talking about professional interest. Talking to reporters is one way to keep up with the issues in your field that are most relevant to the general public. I see it as continuing education.

Recently, I got an e-mail from a reporter asking me to call her to talk about oral cancer screening. I don't know much about oral cancer—it's a relatively rare cause of death. About 8,000 Americans die from it each year. For context, lung cancer kills 160,000—or about twenty times as many. Oral cancer does not even appear in the top ten causes of cancer death; it's number twenty on the list. But I do know something about screening.

The reporter worked for a web portal for dental professionals, one that includes news, features, and columns. I know I said that answering reporters' questions was part of my job. But to be perfectly honest, it does matter who they work for. Those who work for newspapers with names I recognize—be they in New York, LA, Tampa Bay, or Springfield, Illinois—are more likely to get a response than those who work for websites that I've never heard of.

So I was a little hesitant on this one. I wondered if this was really a reporter or someone in public relations. Before I devoted a lot of time I e-mailed her: "Before I call, can you send me any pieces the portal has done questioning dental practices?"

That's my acid-test question. If you can't find any practices to question, it's hard to call it journalism. I got back some stuff on hepatitis and HIV exposure from an oral surgeon (who used rusty instruments and handled needles sloppily) and Medicaid fraud in a Texan dental management company (many of its dentists were performing unnecessary procedures on children—and billing for them). Not exactly what I was looking for—I was hoping for some investigation of routine dental

X-rays (*aren't we all?*)—but I hadn't specified that I was interested in pieces questioning "standard" dental practices. Next time I will.

I called her. She said she was following up on a story in *Consumer Reports* about cancer testing, which said screening for cancers of the bladder, lung, oral cavity, and skin was only necessary in people at high risk. She pointed out this was counter to the American Dental Association and the Oral Cancer Foundation's recommendations that dentists should perform routine screening for oral cancer.

Big surprise. The Oral Cancer Foundation recommends screening for oral cancer. And the American Dental Association—who would do the screening—is totally on board.

Although I had nothing to do with the list in *Consumer Reports*—it comes from the US Preventive Services Task Force—I was quoted in the story. She wanted to know if I thought screening for oral cancer was unnecessary. I started by saying that screening is a more complex topic than it might appear. Many assume screening can only do good. But the truth is that screening is almost certain to produce some harm, while its benefits are more uncertain. She didn't let me get any further than that.

She told me it was simple—and gently suggested that I might not understand. Screening for oral cancer only takes a few minutes and doesn't cost anything extra. There were no harms. She wanted to make sure I understood that advanced oral cancer was a horrible disease (I assured her, I do). Also, that the number of new oral cancer cases is growing among people with no known risk factors like tobacco or alcohol use (I think she even used the word "epidemic"). Survivors agreed that screening was a good thing. So did all the dental experts. There was strong evidence that patients diagnosed with early cancer did much better than those who were diagnosed at later stages.

Wow. In two minutes, she managed to touch every base—every misconception about screening. Misconceptions that always lead to the same answer: more screening. I now understand there was only one right answer to her question: "Yes—everybody should be screened for oral cancer every year."

I don't know what was wrong with me—I am intimately familiar with the single-right-answer question. My wife Linda asks me them from time to time. And I often get them wrong too. By the way, when I related this interview to Linda, she said, *"If she wasn't interested in learning about why there might be an opposing view, why was she calling you?"* I could not answer that.

I wish I could say it was a short call. It wasn't. I wanted to lay out the reasons why we need to be extremely cautious about screening, why we needed reliable data, why finding more cancer wasn't necessarily a good thing, why survival statistics can be so misleading, and why patient anecdotes are not a good information source. She was having none of it.

I should be clear: the perspective of this reporter would have been the typical perspective of health reporters a decade ago. Now more and more of them do understand the subtleties of screening—and the lessons learned from screening for breast and prostate cancer. In fact, I'm probably guilty of assuming that most understand the issue.

So this was a good wake-up call for me: there still is room to improve understanding. The effects of screening remain counterintuitive. And if the reporters don't get it, how can we doctors expect the public to?

WHERE PEOPLE START

A little background: Screening is the systematic search for abnormalities in those who have *no* symptoms of disease. It is a systematic effort to detect disease early.

Your intuition tells you that early detection is the best way to deal with a feared disease like cancer. It feels like prevention—which always sounds like a good thing. We all know that *an ounce of prevention is worth a pound of cure.* That statement is so appealing and so apparently self-evident, that most of us understandably default to: screening is always a good idea.

Because the statement about prevention and cure is so powerful in screening debates, I've been curious about its origins. It's probably an old English proverb. But if you Google it, you will undoubtedly find links attributing it to Ben Franklin. But it wasn't in reference to health:

> In the first Place, as an Ounce of Prevention is worth a Pound of Cure, I would advise 'em to take care how they suffer living Coals in a full Shovel, to be carried out of one Room into another, or up or down Stairs, unless in a Warmingpan shut; for Scraps of Fire may fall into Chinks and make no Appearance until Midnight; when your Stairs being in Flames, you may be forced, (as I once was) to leap out of your Windows, and hazard your Necks to avoid being oven-roasted.

As the creator of one of the first fire departments in the United States, Franklin was interested in preventing fire.

Nonetheless, the idea of prevention is particularly powerful in health. If you want to attribute it to someone, don't think Ben Franklin—think Dick Nixon. It was President Nixon who said, "We need to work out a system that includes a greater emphasis on preventive care." Preventive care was central to his administration's promotion of health maintenance organizations and to the war on cancer. But because the promotion of genuine health—largely dependent upon a healthy diet, exercise, and not smoking—did not fit well in the biomedical culture, preventive care was transformed into a high-tech search for early disease.

Although they are both considered components of preventive medicine (immunization is a third component), it's hard to overstate the magnitude of the gap between health promotion and early disease detection. It's a huge chasm; they are as different as night and day.

Think of health promotion as what your grandmother might have told you when you were young: get plenty of sleep, eat your fruits and vegetables, go play outside—and don't start smoking. Ultimately, as you grew up, the onus was on you to incorporate these behaviors into your lifestyle. Her basic idea was positive: lead a healthy life.

Think of early detection as the effort to find abnormalities—be they structural, biochemical, or even genetic—generally with the assistance of powerful technologies. No one has to make a difficult lifestyle change; instead, health-care professionals do something to you. We take pictures of the inside of your body. We draw your blood and test it for a broad array of molecules. We remove a piece of your tissue and examine it under the microscope. It is a scientific process, a concrete service, and it leads to an "answer." From the doctors' perspective, early detection has other appealing features: ordering a test is quick and easy, and it has an established billing process—unlike health promotion counseling. Not surprisingly, early detection has become the dominant cancer prevention strategy in mainstream American medicine.

But here the basic idea is far less positive: we are looking hard for things to be wrong.

One might argue that early detection should not be considered part of preventive medicine—simply because it is usually not about preventing disease. In fact, the quickest way to get diagnosed with a disease is to be screened for it.

The idea is instead to catch disease early—when presumably it is easier to treat. The intent is to prevent deaths from the disease, just as it is for many of our treatments. But while treatment is focused on a few, screening is dispersed to all.

THE ODDS ARE STACKED AGAINST SCREENING

Historically, doctors directed medical interventions toward people suffering from health problems. That's what the word "patient" used to mean. The problems tended to be readily apparent—in our nomenclature they were "clinically evident." The patients had obvious symptoms, and they had physical manifestations of disease that physicians could objectively observe with their naked eye—what we call "signs" of disease. Treatment was something reserved for that small portion of the population that developed clinically evident disease. In other words, treatment involved a few, all of whom could potentially benefit.

Screening is something done to the entire population: everybody who might get the disease. So screening is up against staggering odds. It must involve many, to potentially benefit a few.

Who might be helped by a population-wide oral cancer screening program? The eight thousand Americans who die from it each year.

Who might be hurt by a population-wide oral cancer screening program? The 240 million American adults who would need to be screened.

Do the math. The ratio of those who could be harmed to those who could be benefited is 30,000:1. That's an uphill battle. There has to be a lot of benefit for the 8,000 and very little harm for the 240 million to be a good trade-off. Of course, not every one of the 240 million will be harmed. But then again, not every one of the 8,000 will be helped. Nevertheless this imbalance—the number who could benefit being so much smaller than the number who could be harmed—makes it very hard for screening to help more than it hurts.

LIMITED BENEFIT: BIRDS IN THE BARNYARD

Let's start with the benefit of cancer screening. It's an important benefit: avoiding a cancer death. At the same time, it's equally important to acknowledge that screening doesn't avoid most cancer deaths. People who are regularly screened still can die from the cancer being screened for. Every randomized trial of screening has shown this. It's not the patient's fault. It's not the doctor's fault. It's not the screening test's fault. Instead it reflects the dynamics of cancer.

When I was in medical school, I was taught that anything labeled "cancer" would inexorably progress. Once a cell had the DNA derangement of cancer, it was only a matter of time until the cancer spread throughout the body. And it was only a matter of time until it killed the patient.

But we now recognize the world of cancer is much more diverse. At one extreme, autopsies have shown that many of us have small cancers that never bother us during life—particularly cancers of the prostate, breast, and thyroid gland. At the other extreme, screening programs have shown that early cancer detection doesn't help everyone; many go on to die from cancer despite early detection. These observations bring us to a new conceptual model of cancer—and to turtles, rabbits, and birds.

It's a barnyard pen of cancers. The goal is not to let any of the animals escape the pen to become deadly. But the turtles aren't going anywhere anyway. They are the indolent, nonlethal cancers. The rabbits are ready to hop out at any time. They are the potentially lethal cancers, cancers that might be stopped by early treatment. Then there are the birds. Quite simply: they are already gone. They are the most aggressive cancers, the ones that have already spread by the time they are detectable, the ones that are beyond cure.

Screening can only help with the rabbits. The turtles don't need help; the birds can't be helped. The turtles create the problem of overdiagnosis (more on that later), the birds create the problem of limited benefit.

Consider this: Despite three decades of widespread screening mammography in the United States, the rate at which women present with metastatic breast cancer is unchanged. That means the number of women who are found to have metastatic breast cancer when they first contact the health system is the same now as it was before we screened for breast cancer (correcting for the size and age composition of the population—as is done for all health statistics).

That's sad. It's not mammography's fault; it's the birds' fault. The birds are the reason that the most favorable findings of randomized trials of screening are on the order of a one-third reduction in the number of cancer deaths. The other two-thirds still die from their cancer—despite screening.

Again, avoiding a cancer death is a really important benefit. But it doesn't happen very often—even in the best of conditions. Imagine a group of one thousand sixty-five-year-old women undergoing screening for breast cancer. Roughly ten of those one thousand women would be expected to die from breast cancer over the next ten years. But screening can't help them all; it might help as many as one-third of them. In other words, it might help around three avoid a cancer death. The number of deaths from prostate cancer—and the number avoided by screening—would be roughly the same for sixty-five-year-old men.

And all that assumes that screening actually reduces the number of cancer deaths by one-third. The most favorable finding for prostate cancer screening was a 20 percent reduction in cancer mortality; the only other major trial showed no reduction in mortality. There have been lots of trials of screening mammography—I'll spare you the details (and refer you to *Should I Be Tested for Cancer?*). The central estimate of its effect is about a 20 percent reduction in cancer mortality. I should be clear that there are a number of us who think that the twenty-to-thirty-year-old trials are no longer relevant since treatment is now so much better. Better treatment makes screening less important. (Why don't we screen for pneumonia? Because treatment for pneumonia is usually so effective.) The advent of adjuvant chemotherapy and hormonal therapy represents a tremendous advance in breast cancer therapy. But our improved ability to treat women who have cancers big enough that they themselves are aware of them (i.e., cancers that are obvious without screening) almost certainly makes screening mammography less useful; my best guess is that mammography now lowers breast cancer mortality by 10 percent—or less.

That's getting pretty small—helping on the order of one per one thousand over ten years. For context, remember that while I'm having a heart attack, running the snake up my groin helps twenty per one thousand—in the next thirty days. One breast surgeon confided to me, "If mammography was a treatment, we'd never do it. The effect is too small."

There are more cancers to screen for than prostate and breast cancer. What do we know about the benefit of other screening tests? Lung cancer screening in heavy smokers with spiral CT: 20 percent reduction in lung cancer mortality. Colon cancer screening with fecal occult blood: 15–33 percent reduction in colon cancer mortality. Liver cancer screening: no effect. Ovarian cancer screening: no effect.

There you have it, that's what we know about benefit. That's why I say the most we can expect from screening is to reduce cancer mortality by about one-third. What limits the benefit? The birds.

And there's a lot of screening going on that hasn't been rigorously studied. Bladder, esophageal, testicular, thyroid, and skin cancer screening—none of these have been studied. Oh, add oral cancer screening to the list.

Why don't we know about the others? Because studying screening is a herculean task. One of my gastroenterology colleagues recently embarked on a randomized trial of colonoscopy screening to determine its effect on colon cancer mortality. Believe it or not, it has never been done. It's another VA Cooperative Study—like the study I described in the first chapter that investigated the effect of treatment in men with really, really high blood pressure during the 1960s. That trial involved 143 men and was completed in less than two years. Doug's colonoscopy trial involves 50,000 patients. He started in 2010; he won't be finished till 2025.

That's a heroic effort. Sometimes I feel a little guilty that I encouraged him to do it.

How can one study be so small and short, while the other has to be so big and long? Because one is testing the effect of focused treatment, while the other is testing the effect of dispersed screening. The hypertension trial examined the effect of treatment in men who would otherwise have a lot of bad things happen to them in the near term (bad things like death, strokes, and heart attacks). In other words, their baseline risk was sky-high. The effect of treatment was huge and could be demonstrated quickly. The colonoscopy trial involves men and women who are well—or, more precisely, don't have colon cancer. Furthermore, the vast majority will never get colon cancer. So investigators have to do colonoscopies on a lot of people to see if it will help the very few destined to get colon cancer.

Like I said, the odds are stacked against screening.

DOES SCREENING SAVE LIVES?

Perhaps you've noticed: I've said nothing about early detection saving lives. Instead, I've written about averting a cancer death, lowering the cancer death rate, and reducing cancer mortality—which are three ways to say the same thing. Saving a life is something different. Screening is often promoted as "saving lives." I bet when most people hear that language they think it means that screening helps people live longer. That's what most of my patients think—and that's what I would have thought before I started to study cancer screening.

The studies of screening make their judgments based on changes in the death rate from the cancer being screened for. In our jargon, they measure cancer-specific mortality. In order for people to "live longer," however, the overall rate of death must fall—deaths from all causes combined. We call that overall or all-cause mortality.

The distinction between cancer deaths and all deaths was highlighted in a recent long-term follow-up of the Minnesota Colon Cancer Control Study—another herculean study of roughly 50,000 people followed for fifteen years. The study was not investigating screening colonoscopy; it was investigating screening for fecal occult blood (a simple test for blood in the stool—often referred to as "stool cards"). Its findings were published in 1993: annual screening reduced colon cancer mortality by 33 percent. It is one of the most influential randomized trials of screening. It's a classic.

In 2013, the investigators published a long-term follow-up: thirty years following the initiation of screening. By now, most of the participants had died; they were between ages fifty and eighty at the start of the study. In the group that wasn't screened, 3 percent died from colon cancer. In the screened group, 2 percent died from colon cancer. In other words, screening reduced the rate of colon cancer death by one-third—that's the 33 percent reduction.

There is a nice graph showing the effect over time. The vertical axis shows the proportion dying from colon cancer, the horizontal axis shows the time from the start of the study: from zero to thirty years. The curve for both groups rises over time as more people die from colon cancer. So even in the screened group, people died from colon cancer. Again, that's the birds. But the curve for the screened group rises more slowly than does the curve for those not screened. At the end of thirty years, the curves end at 2 percent and 3 percent. That's the effect of catching rabbits; that's the benefit of screening.

But there was also a second graph. It too depicted death over time, but in this case it showed the proportion dying for any reason—overall mortality. The curves for the screened group and the not-screened group are right on top of each other. In fact, it just looks like one curve. That means the overall rate of death was exactly the same. Each year the proportion who died was the same for both groups. At the end of thirty years, the curves end at 71 percent and 71 percent. Screening didn't help people live longer. Not even a little bit.

How can that be? Two possible explanations exist: optimistic and pessimistic. The optimistic explanation is chance. While one might expect the overall death curves to end at 70 percent for screening and 71 percent for those not screened—to reflect that 1 percent difference in colon cancer death—by chance it didn't happen that way. The pessimistic explanation is that while screening lowered the rate of death from colon cancer, it also increased the rate of death from other causes. A lot happened to the screening group (tests, procedures, and so on) and a lot of it happened to those not destined to die from colon cancer. Remember: screening must involve many, to potentially help a few. A tiny increase in death among the many could wipe out the larger benefit to the few.

Don't you wish we knew more? Don't you wish we could know for sure that "screening saves lives"?

I can imagine some of my epidemiology professors howling at me.

"Gil, you cannot possibly expect to demonstrate that cancer screening lowers overall mortality! There are simply too few deaths from any particular cancer—and too many deaths from other causes—to ever show that screening actually helps people live longer. The effect of screening on all deaths is expected to be so small, that a study powerful enough to demonstrate it would require hundreds of thousands—perhaps millions—of participants."

All true. But then we should dump the "screening saves lives" language. We should publicly acknowledge that we cannot be sure whether early detection lengthens, shortens, or has no effect on how long people live. And we should be clear that if it takes so many people to find out for sure, then the benefit must be, at best, small.

Or we should suck it up and do the humongous studies.

In case you are wondering, we can say with certainty that some "treatment saves lives." Treatment is different than screening. Remember: treatment involves only a few—the few with disease—all of whom can potentially benefit.

In breast cancer, for example, we can even measure the effect of adding chemotherapy or hormonal therapy to surgical therapy. These interventions lower not only breast cancer mortality; they lower overall mortality. How can we show that patients treated with chemotherapy and/or hormonal therapy live longer—period, end of sentence? Because the patients in the studies all have cancer. Their baseline risk of breast cancer death is high. Breast cancer mortality is a big component—by far the biggest component—of their overall death rate.

There is only one cancer screening test that has definitively been proven to help people live longer: lung cancer screening in heavy smokers. Why? Because heavy smokers face a twenty- to thirty-fold increased risk of lung cancer death. In other words, for heavy smokers, lung cancer is a big component of their overall death rate.

The beneficial effects of population-wide screening are small. Its effect on longevity is uncertain. But no matter how small and uncertain, I believe a few people—on the order of 1 per 1,000—win big. Maybe you are that 1—but you are certainly more likely to be one of the 999. Nevertheless we'd all do it for the chance to be that 1, if nothing bad happened to the others. We'd all do it if there were no harms.

But there are.

SCREENING HARMS—FEAR

Let me start by acknowledging that some of my critics would object to my use of the word "harm" in the next few pages. I warned you there might be some value judgments here. You'll need to decide how you feel about the three adverse outcomes related to screening.

First, to get people interested in screening in the first place we have to get people to worry about the disease we are screening for. The phrase typically used to describe this effort is to "raise awareness." It's a nice euphemism—but it really doesn't describe what needs to be done: some "dis"-ease needs to be introduced into the population. In other words, people need to be scared about dying from the disease; they need to be made to feel more vulnerable.

You may not consider that a harm, but remember health is not simply a state of physical being—it's also a state of mind. It's more than a little ironic for a health-care system to scare people about their health, particularly when we know that doing so can adversely affect their health.

I'm not saying we should never purposely scare people—just that we need to carefully pick and choose. Fear is an integral part of antismoking campaigns. That's appropriate. For those who care about population health, there is nothing more important than reducing the amount of cigarette smoking. There's not only that twenty-to-thirty-fold increase in the most common cause of cancer death in the United States (lung cancer); there's also the doubling in the most common cause of death, period (heart disease), and the virtual certainty that smokers will develop some difficulty breathing if they live long enough. Aside from scaring people, there's no harm to the proposed intervention: stop smoking or, more importantly, don't start.

But fear can backfire—and breast cancer screening is the poster child for the problem. Some women have been made so terrified of the disease, that they are having healthy breasts removed. I'm not referring to Angelina Jolie's decision to have both breasts (and ovaries) removed—she had a rare mutation that dramatically increases the risk of breast and ovarian cancer. I'm referring to women without the mutation, women at average risk for breast cancer. In the United States (and the United Kingdom), about one-quarter of women who develop breast cancer in one breast now ask for both to be removed. A few—to emphasize, a very few—will die from that decision. The thirty-day mortality rate from mastectomy is about a quarter of 1 percent. They will have been literally scared to death.

> There is an enormous climate of fear, whether that's from Breast Cancer Awareness Month or the news media the other 11 months of the year. The only thing you ever hear about breast cancer is about some woman who's dying because she didn't get treated in time.

That's not me talking, that's a breast cancer surgeon—the chief of the Breast Service at Memorial Sloane Kettering. She's worried about scaring women too much.

It is certainly reasonable to ask the question: To what extent should the health-care system be promoting a sense of vulnerability in people who feel well?

SCREENING HARMS—FALSE ALARMS

Second, come back to how the odds are stacked against screening: many (often thousands) must be tested, to potentially benefit a few. Any harms from the testing process—false alarms, complications of diagnostic procedures, etc.—are multiplied since so many people are going through it.

Once again, breast cancer screening is the poster child for the problem. What is most certain about screening mammography in the United States is that it leads to a lot of false alarms: worrisome mammograms, and yet subsequent testing—another mammogram, an ultrasound, an MRI, and/or a biopsy—ultimately finds no cancer. For example, among 1,000 American women age fifty screened annually for a decade, how many will have at least one false alarm? Somewhere between 490 and 670. And 70 to 100 will be biopsied to prove they don't have cancer. These data come from the mammographers themselves—the Breast Cancer Surveillance Consortium—and reflect radiologists with low and high false-alarm rates (25th and 75th percentiles).

A screening program that alarms half the population is outrageous. No European country would tolerate it. Whether you blame the doctors or the system or the malpractice lawyers—it's a problem to be fixed. Reducing false alarms is the primary motivation for changing recommendations from annual to biennial screening.

I can't really do justice to the topic of false alarms following mammography. But the affected women can. When I have a piece pointing out the limitations of mammography in the general press, I get letters like this:

> I am a 66-year-old woman who has had a difficult experience with mammography over the past 20 or so years. For some reason, I have a strong tendency to develop calcifications, most of which they feel the necessity to biopsy. I dread every annual mammogram because the likelihood is very high that something will have to be checked out. So far nothing has been wrong, but I have had one open biopsy and three stereotactic biopsies. The last of those biopsies produced an incidental finding of a papilloma, which they decided to do a "lumpectomy" on because one in ten can hide cancer. The surgery did not go well; they informed me they missed the spot and would have to redo the surgery. Two days later, they decided they had indeed operated on the right area and that there was no cancer in the papilloma. No cancer, but extreme trauma to the patient and a developing panic problem with regard to the whole issue for which I will now be seeing a psychologist.

Or e-mails like this:

> I am a PhD in economics and was able to read the medical literature on the usefulness of biopsies when mammography shows the breast conditions that mine did. I concluded that it was extremely unlikely that I had cancer and, because of illness my husband was facing at the time, I wished to at least postpone the biopsy, but I could not find any support for this decision. All the doctors and nurses I talked with were almost hysterical at the idea that I would not have the biopsy, acting

as though I was giving myself a death sentence. "It's no big deal," they said, "non-invasive." "Nobody gets a second opinion for a biopsy." One of the authors of the most illuminating article I'd seen actually practices in my area and so I thought I'd be able to get support from her. But it turned out to be impossible to consult with her without making an appointment for a biopsy(!).

When I got there, it was like an assembly line. I was stripped and paper-gowned and sent to a waiting room with several other women who were ahead of me. It was obvious that the doctor was someone who had discovered the profit motive since her more-philosophical days when she'd written the article. She said, "Well, probably the best reason to go ahead with the biopsy is that you are here." I don't know why I succumbed at that point, maybe just exhaustion from having to take on the entire medical profession single-handed.

The procedure did not go well; the granules she was looking for were so small that she couldn't find them on the first or second pass. And sticking a 1/2" needle through my breast seemed pretty "invasive" to me. Immediately afterward, they had me get another mammogram which squeezed the band-aid off the wound and caused blood to squirt out. Because of the difficulty in finding the material to biopsy, my breast was bruised badly for weeks on the side opposite where the needle had entered. I used to be someone who went bra-less a good deal of the time, but for the next 5 years, I almost always wore an athletic bra that held my breasts tight against my chest. When the doctor called to tell me the biopsy was negative, she seemed completely unaware of the irony when I said, "Yes, we knew that would be the case, remember?" Since I never want to be in that vulnerable situation again, I have not had another mammogram.

I think the screening culture has had a tendency to downplay the problem of false alarms—even trivialize the discomfort and anxiety by juxtaposing it with the need to "save lives." But it matters. Maybe it goes without saying: fear and pain is not good for human health. Medical care needs to work on reducing psychological stress—not creating it.

A number of women have told me they stopped mammography because they got so tired, frustrated, scared, or angry about false alarms. And recent research has documented that the psychological effects—anxiety, negative impact on sexuality and sleep, loss of inner calm—persist for at least three years following a false alarm. Of course, it doesn't affect every woman the same way. Some may initially fear for their life only to be told a few days later that everything is fine. They are thankful and may even feel that the experience has given them some important new perspective on life. Others are left in limbo. While told they don't have cancer, they are not told that everything is fine. Instead they learn their breasts are somehow abnormal—that they have dysplasia or atypia, that they are at "high risk"—and can only worry because the doctors aren't doing anything about it. Nothing, except more mammograms.

SCREENING HARMS—OVERDIAGNOSIS

Finally, screening produces the harm of overdiagnosis. While the term sounds like it simply means "excessive diagnosis," it has a more precise definition in cancer screening. Overdiagnosis occurs when a cancer is diagnosed, yet the cancer is not destined to cause symptoms or death. Overdiagnosis does not imply misdiagnosis: the cellular abnormality found does, in fact, meet the pathologic criteria for cancer. And overdiagnosis should not be confused with a false alarm: patients with false alarms are told they don't have cancer and *are not* treated; overdiagnosed patients are told that they do have cancer and *are* treated.

Whenever doctors screen for cancer we end up treating a lot more people than we would otherwise. We look hard for early forms of cancer, we find more "cancer," and we treat more "cancer." By now you are surely wondering: What does that word mean? Dr. George Crile—a cancer surgeon at the Cleveland Clinic—thinks about it this way:

> In clinical practice, to say that a person has cancer gives as little information about the possible course of his disease as to say that he has an infection. There are dangerous infections that may be fatal and

there are harmless infections that are self-limited or may disappear. The same is true of cancers. Cancer is not a single entity. It is a broad spectrum of diseases related to each other only in name.

Amazingly, that statement appeared on the pages of *Life* magazine in 1955—the year I was born—a rude reminder that I've never had an original idea in my life. Crile may, in fact, be the originator of the barnyard-pen analogy—although I can't confirm that. I can confirm, however, that Crile would definitely get the turtle problem: the cancers that aren't going anywhere anyway.

It's the turtles that make overdiagnosis possible. Practically speaking, we only find turtles by screening. (A cancer that becomes clinically evident—because of either signs or symptoms—is, by definition, not a turtle.) But screening also identifies some rabbits and few birds. Since we doctors cannot reliably distinguish which animal is which, we treat them all—"just to be safe." That means screening leads us to treat turtles. If your cancer is a turtle, however, you can't be helped by treatment—because there is nothing to fix. But you can be hurt by treatment. Finding and treating turtles: that's the problem of overdiagnosis and overtreatment.

You want a feel for the problem? You want narrative? It would go something like this:

I am a middle-aged [pick one: woman/man] who was encouraged to participate in [pick one: breast/prostate] cancer screening by [pick one: my hospital, my health plan, a television news story, a radio "public service announcement," an advertisement, a celebrity, or a sportscaster]. My screening led to the detection of a small cancer for which I received [select from a menu of combinations: surgery, hormonal therapy, chemotherapy, radiation]. Because of complications from my therapy, I do not feel as well now as I did before this whole thing started. Imagine how angry I became to learn I went through all this for nothing—my cancer was not going anywhere anyway.

Of course, that's a fictional narrative. Nonfiction versions are rare. That's because once someone has been treated, no one knows for sure who has been overdiagnosed. We know some have—because we are treating so many more than would ever develop clinically evident cancer—we just don't know which ones. But the new patients understandably choose to see themselves as having benefited—they see themselves as survivors. The absence of compelling patient stories about overdiagnosis means the idea remains unfamiliar to the general public, but it doesn't mean the harm is any less real.

When it comes to overdiagnosis, prostate cancer screening is the poster child. There are a whole lot of prostate cancer turtles. And the older men get, the more turtles there are. By age sixty, over half of men are found to have small prostate cancers on autopsy—even though they will have died from something else. Screening doesn't find all of these small cancers, but it finds a lot of them. And when a prostate cancer is found, the primary treatment is to remove the prostate.

No one wants unneeded treatment. But unneeded removal of the prostate is particularly problematic. I'm not saying that because of my sex; I'm saying that because of human anatomy. The prostate gland sits deep in the pelvis. It's wrapped around the urethra—the tube that drains urine from the bladder to the penis—and wrapped around it are nerves en route to the penis. Suffice it to say, the prostate was not designed for easy removal.

Guys, think of it like removing the heater core in your car. It's not easy to get to either. You gotta take the dash off and that means disconnecting a lot of vacuum lines and electrical wires. If you need help, check out the "how to replace a heater core" videos on YouTube. A comment on one video captured the challenge nicely: "*I'd rather start a small controlled fire in the car for heat each time I drove it in the winter instead of attempting this.*"

To be fair, the surgeons have gotten reasonably good at it. Nevertheless, somewhere around half of men will have some complication following the procedure. These complications reflect the underlying anatomy: plumbing problems (leaking or difficult with urination) and electrical problems (sexual dysfunction).

I was reminded of one other problem to consider when I ran into a colleague at our local recycling center (which, here in the People's Republic, serves as the major venue for social interactions). Bob told me about a friend who was screened for prostate cancer, found to have it, and then underwent surgery. Following surgery, he had a blood clot go to his lungs and died. He was fifty-eight (that's my age, margin of error: ± 2 years). So the effort to address a finding that may—or may not—become a problem in the future, leads to a death that happens now.

Anesthesia, surgery, and a period of bedridden recovery can all combine to produce life-threatening complications. I want to be clear: this happens rarely—the thirty-day mortality rate from prostatectomy is about one-half of 1 percent (and lower for minimally invasive prostatectomy). But just because it happens rarely, doesn't mean that it doesn't happen.

Overdiagnosis and overtreatment is very common in prostate cancer screening. In the twenty-plus years of screening, it's happened to more than a million American men. Roughly half have suffered a plumbing or electrical problem from treatment for a cancer that was never going to bother them. And a few, a very few, have died. But screening doesn't discriminate based on sex: in the thirty-plus years of breast cancer screening, more than a million American women have been overdiagnosed and overtreated.

The morbidity and complications of unneeded cancer treatment represent the major harm of overdiagnosis. However, two other observations are worth mentioning. First, the emotional burden of cancer diagnosis can be overwhelming for a few: cancer patients face an increased risk of suicide (even among low-risk prostate cancer patients). Second, the financial burden of a cancer diagnosis is overwhelming for many: cancer patients face an increased risk of bankruptcy. Two more reasons to think twice about looking for turtles.

Your intuition might suggest that there is no downside to looking for early forms of cancer—it can only help. But this intuition is wrong.

Arguably, the opposite is more plausible: there is no upside—it can only hurt. Think of what needs to happen for a screening test to even have a chance of working for the few it could help. Everyone must be made concerned enough to get screened, everyone must be tested, many retested and needlessly alarmed, while others are overdiagnosed and overtreated.

In other words: it's the harms that are certain, not the benefits.

THE FINAL BLOW: THE TYRANNY OF PERFORMANCE

There has been a long-standing subculture in medicine interested in improving the quality of health care. Who can argue with that? Simultaneously, there has been an increased interest in measurement: to carefully document what is actually happening out there. I'm part of that subculture—so, of course, I think it's a good thing.

The problem arises when the two subcultures converge to attempt to measure quality. While this is conceptually straightforward, the operational details get fuzzy quickly. Though we might be able to agree about what true quality is—a doctor who takes the time to figure out what is going on with you, has the skills to make the right diagnosis and treatment plan, works as part of a system that can reliably carry out that plan, and is both supportive and able to meet your needs as you heal—the problem is that these attributes are not readily apparent in the electronic medical record. Furthermore, different doctors will have different definitions of what constitutes "the right diagnosis and treatment plan," and different patients will have different definitions of what constitutes "supportive and able to meet your needs." True quality is extremely hard to measure.

What is easy to measure is whether doctors do things. Doing things generates a bill; a bill generates electronic data. All the combined culture of quality-plus-measurement needed was to identify things that doctors should do to every patient. Things that everyone agreed were important to people's health. Like screening.

Let the PhD economist—whose breast biopsy "did not go well," who never wanted to "be in that vulnerable situation again," who did not want another mammogram—take it from here:

> I joined Kaiser a few years ago, foolishly thinking that they would be more in agreement with my own minimalist attitude toward all things medical. The nurse in my doctor's office harassed me for months, e-mailing me and calling my home phone and my cell, leaving messages, pleading with me to get a mammogram and implying that my failure to do so would almost guarantee that I will die of breast cancer. This continued despite me explaining clearly to both the doctor and nurse my reasons for not getting a mammogram. I finally changed doctors (within Kaiser) and have had no more phone calls. But I'm sure it is as you say in the article, that Kaiser too is using the number of mammograms as a measure of "quality of care."

Persistent e-mails and phone calls after declining a mammogram? That's not quality; that's harassment. Suggesting that her decision will lead to breast cancer death? That's not quality; that's intimidation (not to mention fraud).

OK. Now I have to do something I don't like to do: criticize what I think is otherwise one of our better health-care systems—Kaiser Permanente (a large prepaid group practice originally created as a way to provide medical care to workers and their families at the largest construction site in history—the Grand Coulee Dam). It's the same way I feel when I criticize my former employer of many years: the VA. Because both systems depend on salaried physicians, both provide a healthy alternative to the excesses of fee-for-service medicine. Both have a laudable interest in delivering quality care; both have created undesirable side effects in their effort to do so.

The problem is the blunt performance measure: one in which doing something is always the right answer. To be fair, the performance measures typically come from a higher level—such as the National Committee for Quality Assurance. But, to be equally fair, both systems have chosen to sign on to them—rather than question them.

Screening mammography was one of the original performance measures for comprehensive health-care systems: one grade on a "health care report card" first created during the early 1990s. Kaiser wants to perform well; Kaiser wants to get good grades.

A few years ago, *Health Affairs* asked me to review a manuscript detailing Kaiser's efforts to improve mammography performance. It described interventions to reduce the wait time for a mammogram, strategies to maximize each machine's "throughput," mechanisms to "give credit" to primary care physicians (including small financial incentives for physician groups) or mechanisms to hold them "accountable," the development of new electronic data systems to prompt mammography, and efforts to contact women via both a letter and an automated phone contact. That's right: robocalls.

It went on to detail the discovery of another approach to "maintain the energy and focus on improving (screening) rates"—the power of patient stories. They made a video of one woman whose "breast cancer was detected early after a receptionist in Ophthalmology persistently encouraged her to get a mammogram, *despite the woman's continued reluctance to do so.*"

That's not quality; that's a violation of medicine's fundamental ethical principle: patient autonomy. While there may be a public health imperative to screen selected populations (e.g., doctors) for selected infectious diseases (e.g., tuberculosis), that's because an infection in one individual affects the chance of it developing in another. But that is not the case for chronic disease: my having cancer doesn't affect your risk of cancer.

Cancer screening is not a public health imperative, it is a choice. The reason is that it is a close call: a delicate balance of benefits and harms that different individuals—facing the same situation—can rationally make different decisions about based on their values and preferences.

TURTLES MAKE SCREENING LOOK GOOD

Ironically our cancer statistics tend to hide the close-call reality and paint a rosy picture instead. It's the turtles' fault. Here's how it works.

Because of the existence of turtles, screening finds more cancers than would otherwise be found. This shows up in our statistics as higher cancer incidence rates—the number of cancers diagnosed per million people. This worrisome rise in incidence leads to calls for more screening. That's misleading, because we are inevitably finding more and more turtles that have always been there.

But what is much more misleading is that now the typical cancer patient does much better. This shows up as higher survival rates—the proportion of cancer patients who are alive five or ten years after diagnosis. That's really misleading: just by finding more cancers not destined to cause death, it looks like something really good is happening. Of course survival rates go up if you add in patients with cancers that were never going anywhere anyway. Screening gets credit for curing turtles.

I know how to design a blockbuster screening test. Have it find cancer in everybody. In a few months, I'll be able to legitimately say we have a new cancer epidemic on our hands. A few years later, I'll point out that the survival rates are damn near 100 percent. All thanks to me.

Statistics can be mind-numbing. A lot of folks respond better to narrative. Luckily turtles not only make great statistics, they make great stories. The turtles make for powerful witnesses—cancer survivors—that constitute perhaps the most misleading information in all of medicine. Everyone has heard survivor stories on the news; increasingly many of us have a more personal exposure: a coworker, a neighbor, a friend, or a family member. Nowhere is that more true than in breast and prostate cancer.

As I write this, Amy Robach has just announced she has breast cancer. She is an anchor for *Good Morning America*. As part of breast cancer awareness month, the forty-year-old had her first mammogram—on morning television. A month later, in front of five million viewers, she announced that she had cancer and said, "Having a mammogram saved my life."

That's powerful. Who can argue with that?

But what we don't know about Ms. Robach—or our coworker, neighbor, friend, or family member—is whether she actually benefited from early detection. It is entirely possible that she and others would have done just as well had their cancer been diagnosed following the appearance of signs and symptoms. It's also possible they were overdiagnosed: the cancer was never destined to kill them or even make them sick.

Let's give screening the benefit of the doubt. Ignore the question of whether it truly "saves lives"; simply assume it does. Now compare the number of lives saved to the number overdiagnosed. In its pamphlet to help women decide about mammography screening in the United Kingdom, the National Health Service now explicitly tells women their chance of overdiagnosis is about three times higher than their chance of avoiding a breast cancer death. That makes the "lives saved to overdiagnosed ratio" 1:3.

Note these are the numbers from the folks who run—and who promote—the screening program. They are basing their lives saved data on twenty-to-thirty-year-old trials that likely overestimate the benefit of screening, and their overdiagnosis data are based on UK diagnostic practice—which is more prudent than US practice. Given current conditions, my estimate of the ratio in the United States is closer to 1:10.

Everyone agrees overdiagnosis is a bigger problem for prostate cancer screening. There are simply more turtles in the prostate. The most favorable "lives saved to overdiagnosed ratio" here is 1:30. The more pessimistic is 1:100.

Sorry, that's a lot of ratios: 1:3, 1:10, 1:30, 1:100. But they all have one thing in common: more people are on the overdiagnosed side.

Now think about a survivor story following breast or prostate cancer screening. The standard explanation is that her or his life was "saved" by screening. As you can now see, however, the much more likely explanation is that she or he was overdiagnosed. So what is happening is that one of the harms of screening is being misinterpreted as a benefit.

Finding turtles is harmful; don't give us credit for curing them.

CIRCLING BACK TO ORAL CANCER

So what would oral cancer screening look like? The first step will be to raise awareness about oral cancer. That campaign should be straight-forward: the eight thousand deaths a year is as good a place as any to start—but don't provide any context by saying anything about the nineteen competing cancers that are a more common cause of death. Superimpose the body count message on a few high-res photos of some advanced—and preferably, particularly gruesome—oral cancers. Say nothing about their strong relationship to heavy alcohol exposure and cigarette smoking—that would narrow the audience too much. And it goes without saying: simply assert (or at least imply) that screening will help.

Teach the dentists how to examine everyone thoroughly. They'll need some better equipment: we can't trust their fingers and naked eyes. Special lights will help, special stains and mouthwashes, maybe even immunofluorescence, and, of course, special biopsy tools. Lots of opportunities for device manufacturers here.

The dentists will start on their regular patients at first, some of whom will not even know they are being screened. The American Dental Association may even make oral cancer screening a performance measure for their current patients. The dentists will quickly see that it is in their interest to extend screening more broadly. They will offer free screening days, knowing that their long-term effect will be more repeat examinations and more biopsies—neither of which will be free. The oral surgeons will quickly have more cancers to operate on. Some of the operations won't go so well.

My tribe—the epidemiologists—will soon note that the incidence of oral cancer (and oral pre-cancer) is rising. Some will be worried and someone, somewhere, will play the epidemic card. Websites will pick it up, and so will Dr. Oz and the rest of the medical self-help and infotain-ment industry. There will be some voices urging caution, but they will be government or academic types and their messaging clumsy at best. Keep it simple, stupid: early detection saves lives.

At this point, people will start worrying about canker sores in their mouth.

And then the coup de grace: the survivor stories will appear. Someone famous will have their oral cancer caught early and will become a spokesman for the effort. Oral cancer survival rates start going up—providing the scientific proof that good things are happening.

Is anything good happening? Perhaps, but I'm certainly not sure. Is anything bad happening? You tell me. And if you think this is too fanciful, you should know this scenario is what played out in prostate cancer screening.

A NEW CONCEPTUAL MODEL

Maybe I'm painting too pessimistic a picture. More and more people get that screening is more complicated than it appears at first blush. More people understand that early forms of cancer are more common than advanced forms. More appreciate that treatments often produce problems. More grasp how misleading survivors—and survival statistics—can be. And more and more of these people are doctors in the field. They increasingly recognize that cancer screening is a choice, not a public health imperative.

And cancer researchers really are looking at cancer differently. They understand the barnyard pen of cancer—and are even considering adding another animal to it. It turns out that some cellular abnormalities that meet the pathological definition of cancer will go away on their own. Disappear. Regress. Become extinct. Call them the dodos.

Dodos were first recognized in a rare cancer of young children: neuroblastoma. These cancers, which generally start near the kidney, make adrenaline-like substances. Some grow as large as a grapefruit (which in an infant is huge), some invade major blood vessels (like the aorta), and some metastasize to major organs (like the liver). Some are birds, while others go away.

The dodos were recognized when doctors explored screening for neuroblastoma. The doctors found more infants had the cancer than they expected and worried that they were treating too many infants with surgery and chemotherapy. So they simply observed some infants with small cancers. No treatment at all. And their cancers disappeared. The dodo phenomenon has been observed in other cancers: renal cell carcinoma, melanoma, even early breast cancer.

This gets geneticists thinking in a new way. They have been frustrated that detailing a cancer's genetics wasn't more help—that, for many cancers, no single genotypic "marker" provided a dominant, reproducible signal of "badness" or "goodness." In short, the genes in a cancer often can't reliably distinguish between the birds, rabbits, turtles, and dodos.

I went to a conference with a bunch of cancer geneticists a few years back. There were presentations on sequencing, structural rearrangements, microarrays, multiple clones, and genomic instability. Some of it was tough sledding for me, but I did get their frustration: if the question was cancer, the genome wasn't the answer. Then there was a presentation on zebra mussels.

Zebra mussels? The invasive mollusk that infested the Great Lakes and now clogs the intake pipes of water treatment and power plants? It was a great story—I was particularly fascinated by how they had spread from the Caspian Sea in the ballast water of ocean-going ships—but what the hell did zebra mussels have to do with cancer?

Because the next basic science of cancer is ecology. The presentation was given by an oncologist/cancer biologist who wanted to know what the conditions needed to be for a cancer to metastasize—say from the Caspian Sea to the Great Lakes. He argued that it was increasingly apparent that the lethality of a cancer is not simply a function of the cancer itself but also something about the environment in which the cancer lives—the host environment. He articulated an emerging view that the reductionist approach—learning more and more about the fine structure of cancers (from the individual cells to the genetic code within them)—was too narrow. Researchers needed to consider the ecology of cancer.

Oddly enough, Sir David Smithers, a radiotherapist in London, presaged this view in 1962:

> Cancer is no more a disease of cells than a traffic jam is a disease of cars. A lifetime of study of the internal-combustion engine would not help anyone understand our traffic problems.

I get it: You can't learn much about what causes gridlock by studying the fine structure of piston clearance. The title of one of Dr. Smithers's articles captures it all: no cell is an island.

Understanding cancer requires understanding the human ecosystem. Reducing cancer burden is undoubtedly more about keeping that ecosystem healthy, not devising new ways to find smaller and smaller collections of wayward cells.

PRESCRIPTION: ASK FOR DATA—ABOUT BOTH BENEFITS AND HARMS—AND KNOW IT'S A CHOICE

When considering screening, recall the general principles. Many must be involved, to potentially benefit a few. Harms are expected: false alarms are a certainty; some degree of overdiagnosis—and overtreatment—is likely.

I'm not saying screening is always the wrong thing to do. (I believe we all should know something about our blood pressure and weight, but whether that requires screening is a separate question.) Instead I'm saying that because screening may cause you some harm, you have to make sure not only that it produces some benefit—but that it produces *sufficient* benefit to warrant accepting the possible harms.

The first question to ask is obvious: Is there good evidence of benefit? Good evidence means a randomized trial showing lower cancer mortality, not observations crediting turtles with higher survival rates. Frequently, the honest answer will be no. If so, I'd stop there. If benefit hasn't been proven, I wouldn't pursue the test—because harms are always part of the deal.

If there is evidence of benefit, the decision gets more complicated. Now it's a gamble. Ideally, you would like some numbers. How many benefit? How many are harmed? Remember the benefit is a big win—avoiding a cancer death—but it is rare. You need to decide how you feel about the uncertainty in the "saving lives" language, the uncertainty about all-cause mortality. Consider how you value the harm of overdiagnosis and overtreatment relative to the benefit of avoiding a cancer death—knowing that this harm is generally more frequent than the benefit. Finally, you also need to decide how you feel about the much more common—but arguably much less important—harm of false alarms.

In case it helps, here's how I think about prostate cancer screening. I believe that it does help a few men avoid a prostate cancer death—on the order of one per one thousand men my age (I'm close to sixty) over the next ten years. The overdiagnosis and overtreatment problem is much more common—on the order of, at least, thirty per one thousand over the same period. Sexual and urinary function is something I value highly—even if these functions are compromised in only ten of those thirty, I'd say it's a bad deal. Ten times more likely to have an unnecessary sexual or urinary problem than avoid a cancer death? I don't even need to factor in the false alarm and biopsy problems.

And although I'd say the call is closer for mammography—because overdiagnosis is not as common and overtreatment not as morbid—I believe I would ultimately come to the same judgment were I a woman.

But that's me. I tend to mark down the benefit of screening because it happens in the future, while the harms are much more immediate. Avoiding death isn't my top priority anyway; I'd rather avoid a lingering cognitive decline in a long-term care facility (not that I'm likely to be successful). And I place considerable value on not having my life become medicalized—until my symptoms demand it.

You may well choose to be screened. For a small group of individuals the screening deal is much better: those at very high risk of dying from the cancer being sought—and those at a relatively low risk of dying from something else. But even those at average risk can look at the same numbers and come to an equally rational conclusion: they may choose to be screened.

If you do choose screening, here's one idea to help minimize the harms: take your time. What should you do if your screening test is a bit abnormal? Take your time. Often the best strategy is simply to repeat it in six months. Time has real diagnostic value. What should you do if you are found to have early cancer? Take your time. We have overstated the need to act quickly. Find out the options. Get second opinions—an independent opinion—not one from someone who is almost certainly bound to echo the first.

Finally, while the chapter was focused on cancer screening, know that these principles apply to screening in general. There's a lot of screening out there: carotid artery screening, coronary artery screening, abdominal aortic aneurysm screening—and that's just for your arteries. When we screen, we always find more, treat more, and treat some needlessly.

The truth is, screening is a mixed bag. There will be winners and losers. It makes more sense for some diseases than others and it makes more sense for some individuals than others. But it should always be an informed choice.

IT NEVER HURTS TO GET MORE INFORMATION

Disturbing truth: Data overload can scare patients and distract your doctor from what's important

IN THIS CHAPTER I'M GOING to argue that more information is not always better.

It sounds so anti-science. Like I want to live in a world where we accept that the sun revolves around the earth, man's advent on the planet occurs twenty-four hours following the appearance of all other living creatures, and the earth's continents are each fixed in place.

I don't. Science has always been my favorite subject. In fact, I'm auditing an undergraduate course in environmental science as I write this—yesterday featured atmospheric circulation and how the Hadley cells move north and south with the thermal equator. I thought it was fascinating.

I'm a data guy. Most of my research involves analysis of publicly available data. If I'm working, you can bet a spreadsheet is open at some point of the day. And just like every other researcher of my generation, I am frequently reminded how the information age has transformed our work. I can remember trips to the library, descending into some deep dark basement to an area labeled "Government Documents," and then going on a treasure hunt for the relevant massive bound volume hidden somewhere in the stacks (or worse yet, having the hunt involve fiddling around on a microfiche reader). I would then copy the data by hand—and then enter them by hand into a rudimentary desktop computer. The ability to access the world's data from virtually anywhere on the planet represents a quantum leap.

And I think we need more information. In particular, I am a strong advocate for obtaining more information about the effects of medical interventions—information on the full range of effects, with attention to both the benefits and harms.

But I'm not particularly interested in more information about myself. (After this chapter's introduction, I suspect you feel the same way.) Here I'm referring to clinical information: information specific to one individual. Some might call it biometrics—detailed data on the anatomic, physiologic, biochemical, or genetic status of me. While I can imagine some plausible benefits of this kind of information for those of us who are well, it is much easier for me to imagine its harms. More on this later.

For those with symptoms, clinical information is typically viewed as unambiguously useful. That's why we doctors order so many tests. Without a doubt, diagnostic tests can be invaluable in sorting out what is wrong and what to do about it. But they can also be confusing, distracting, and anxiety provoking. Clinical information is a double-edged sword—and physicians are having to sort through more and more of it.

MR. BAKER'S UNNECESSARY DISTRACTION

Let me start at the end of this story. Mr. Baker was on the autopsy table. I was an extremely interested observer: he had been my patient for the previous fifteen years. The pathologist found that he had died from a massive pneumonia. But I wasn't interested in how he died. There was no mystery there—he had been on a ventilator in the intensive care unit for the previous week. I was interested in his kidney.

Mr. Baker and I had worried about his kidney for the previous decade. I hate to say this, but this kidney had become the focus of his care. Despite the fact he had more pressing urinary and vascular problems, we talked about it every visit, and every six months I ordered an abdominal CT scan to check up on it. Why? Because we knew he had kidney cancer.

How could anything be more pressing than a cancer? Because this cancer was a turtle—it had never bothered him during his life. Check that: the only thing that bothered him was the fact that we had found it. The only thing that bothered him was the information.

The autopsy confirmed that he had kidney cancer. More importantly, it confirmed the cancer was a turtle—it had not spread to the lungs, to the liver, to the brain, or anywhere beyond the kidney. Ten years of concern and twenty-some scans in response to one piece of information. You could characterize it as useless information; you could characterize it as harmful information. You be the judge.

Root-cause analyses are quite the vogue in medicine—so let's go back to how the cancer had been discovered a decade earlier. It's a classic medical cascade: in which one event begets another. Mr. Baker had been hoarse for six weeks. Given the duration—and the lack of other symptoms—I sent him to our ear, nose, and throat doctor. He saw a growth on Mr. Baker's left vocal cord and removed it, and the hoarseness resolved. That should have been the end of the story, except someone ordered a chest X-ray to check for lung cancer. To be sure, lung cancer can cause hoarseness, but we had already found an explanation for Mr. Baker's hoarseness. Although the likelihood of having two independent explanations for the same symptom is extremely small, the likelihood that people entering our medical-care system undergo testing of questionable utility is extraordinarily high. Just to check things out.

There was no lung cancer on Mr. Baker's chest X-ray. But there was an abnormality: the space between his two lungs was wider than normal. The radiologist thought we should check that out with a chest CT scan. The chest CT showed that nothing was wrong with that space; in fact, the entire chest was normal. But to capture the entire chest, the scan had to include a little of Mr. Baker's abdomen. And there was the kidney cancer.

Hoarseness leads to kidney cancer. Not in terms of disease progression, mind you. Instead, in terms of medical-care progression: a cascade of events driven by the desire to "be sure" and the assumption that it never hurts to get more information.

Mr. Baker would argue with that assumption.

So would more and more doctors. They are intimately familiar with the problem exemplified in Mr. Baker's story. As we try to amass more information about a patient's symptoms, we increase the chance of stumbling onto something else. We even have a name for the things we stumble onto: incidentalomas.

It would have been easier on me—and perhaps even on Mr. Baker—if we had just taken his kidney out. Problem solved. Of course, solving one problem has a way of begetting another. Like death—about 2 percent of patients Mr. Baker's age die within thirty days of an operation to remove the kidney. Like renal failure—about 10 percent develop chronic kidney disease after the operation, a risk that would undoubtedly have been higher for Mr. Baker since his unaffected kidney was quite small. The irony is that, had the operation been done and bad things had happened, many would view the collateral damage as being acceptable given the overriding goal of curing a cancer.

But we now know this cancer didn't need to be cured. It was a turtle.

You might have thought that stumbling onto something—particularly something labeled "cancer"—could only be a good thing. But understanding turtles and knowing Mr. Baker's story, now you can see that it can be a bad thing. My bet is that the net effect of information provided by incidental detection is harm: it creates too much unnecessary anxiety and too many unneeded procedures.

But I can't prove that. There has never been a randomized trial of the value of incidental detection, nor is it likely there ever will be. It's tough to randomize someone into an intervention that leads to a lot of incidental findings—although not impossible, a randomized trial of conventional colonoscopy (involving a fiber optic device that only "sees" the inside of the colon) versus virtual colonoscopy (involving a CT scan that "sees" all the other organs in the abdomen as well) would do the trick. But randomized trials that speak to the value of more information do exist.

THREE TRIALS ON THE VALUE OF INFORMATION

Consider three trials testing three very different levels of information-gathering in patients with medical problems. The first gathered information very expansively, basically looking for anything wrong. I'd call it a shotgun approach—maybe even a sawed-off shotgun. The second examined the value of a single piece of physiologic information. While this would be a rifle using the foregoing analogy, it's really better labeled as a laser. The third is somewhere in between: seeking multiple pieces of information all directed at the same question. Since I'm already guilty of mixing metaphors, consider it a flashlight.

Enhanced communication: First the shotgun—another VA Cooperative Study, like the hypertension and colonoscopy trials. The study subjects were 1,400 veterans in the hospital because of diabetes, lung disease, or heart disease. They were severely ill patients—the type of patients who, after discharge from the hospital, frequently must be readmitted. Roughly one-half were expected to be readmitted in the next six months. The goal of this study was to reduce that number.

Half of the patients were randomized to standard care; half were randomized to what was called an "intensive primary care intervention." The intervention was not a drug, nor was it a procedure—it was a series of organizational changes to enhance information flow. Before being discharged, patients in the intervention group met with their primary care physician and nurse. They reviewed what had happened during the hospitalization and the proposed changes to the medication regimens. They also assessed the patients' post-discharge needs, provided educational materials, and made post-discharge plans. The nurses called each patient within two days of discharge, and the physicians saw each patient within a week. The patients were given enhanced access to their doctors—including the ability to page them for a phone call. The intervention designed to enhance communication—the flow of unspecified information—between patients and their caregivers.

How could that not be good?

It wasn't. In the investigators' own words, "The effect of our intervention on hospital use was contrary to that predicted by our hypothesis." In normal language, the intervention failed spectacularly. What was the effect of all that additional information? More readmission to the hospital. For the statisticians: significantly more.

There was no evidence that the extra hospitalization helped patients. There was no improvement in their self-assessed health status. There was no reduction in their rate of death—which was, in fact, a little higher in the intervention group, although this probably was due to chance.

So what went wrong? To be honest, no one knows for sure. But I can weave a story. The intervention gave both the primary care nurse and the physician a greater opportunity to seek information about potential problems. Knowing the purposes of the study led the providers to pursue these problems in greater depth. Intervention patients had 70 percent more clinic visits than controls and had an average of seven phone calls (controls had none). The providers sought information more often, sought information in greater depth, and found more problems. And once potential problems were found, it was hard not to do something—something that had the potential to be harmful. In other words, the study intervention resulted in clinical cascades: more potential problems identified, more diagnostic testing, more diagnosis, more treatment, and more hospitalization. In short, the additional information produced problems.

Lung impedance: Now consider a randomized trial of information focused like a laser: gathering a single physiologic—in fact, electrical—variable. To get what is going on requires a little knowledge of the underlying disease process . . . and a little physics. So buckle your seat belt.

Congestive heart failure is one of the most common reasons for hospital admission. The term refers to a chronic condition in which the heart muscle is unable to pump blood adequately. It can happen for a number of reasons, but coronary artery disease (described earlier, in chapter 2) is by far the most common. When the heart can't keep up with its workload, fluid accumulates upstream on both sides of the pump: upstream of the right half (the body) and upstream of the left half (the lungs). Fluid accumulation produces symptoms that lead patients to the hospital: extra fluid in the body causes swelling (particularly in the feet and ankles), extra fluid in the lungs causes shortness of breath.

Congestive heart failure is also one of the most common reasons for hospital readmission. Patients with heart failure are admitted so frequently that they are dubbed "frequent fliers" in medical slang.

Consequently, there has been great interest—some might say excessive interest—in reducing the frequency of hospital readmission among heart failure patients. A common line of inquiry has been to seek early signs of fluid accumulation. The idea is that patients demonstrating these signs could receive prompt pharmacologic intervention to reduce the amount of fluid—and the chance of hospitalization.

The conventional sign of fluid accumulation is a rapid increase in the patient's weight. That's why, in heart failure patients, we doctors are so focused on daily weights. But since other things affect day-to-day weight, there has been a considerable effort given to a more direct measure of fluid accumulation—in particular, within the organ in which excess fluid is most worrisome: the lung.

The advent of implantable cardiac devices—pacemakers and defibrillators—provided the opportunity to make a more direct measurement. These devices have electrodes in the heart muscle and, roughly half a foot away, a battery pack underneath the skin near the collarbone. It didn't require a quantum leap in technology to measure the electrical impedance between the two—in effect measuring the resistance of the upper portion of the lung. Water conducts electricity better than air. In other words, water provides less electrical impedance than air. So if there is a lot of air in the lung, impedance will be high; if there is a lot of fluid, impedance will be low.

Any questions? Or have you had enough physics for the day?

The real question is: Does this information help patients stay out of the hospital? In 2011, the cardiology journal *Circulation* published a randomized trial addressing this question. All of the patients had heart failure and all had implantable defibrillators with the capability of measuring lung impedance. The randomization simply determined whether that capability was turned on—or not.

The primary effect of more information was again more hospitalization—about 80 percent more hospitalizations for heart failure. That's not what the investigators were looking for. And there was no evidence that the hospitalizations helped patients. The patients with more information, again, actually died slightly more often—although, again, this is probably the result of chance.

One thing was very certain: more information had patients coming to the clinic more often—about three times as often as those with the impedance measurement function turned off. Why? Because those who had their impedance monitored could recognize when their impedance fell. When this happened, the article detailed, the patients were "alerted . . . with an audible tone."

I'd call that an alarm, wouldn't you?

Why were these patients coming to see the doctor so often? Because they had alarms going off inside of them. Alarms that didn't help—they were made to worry unnecessarily. The author of the accompanying editorial summed it up nicely in his title, "Too Much Information."

Can you hear Siri on your new iPhone impedance monitor?

"Your lung is now filling with fluid . . ."

Measuring lung impedance and facilitating patient-provider communication represent opposite ends of the information spectrum—from a single variable of electrical conductivity to a wide-open channel of multiple, unspecified variables. But both produced the same result: more unneeded medical care.

I always like the middle ground; maybe the flashlight will work better.

Cancer metastases: The third trial investigated whether women would benefit from intensive diagnostic follow-up after treatment of breast cancer. Most breast cancers don't spread elsewhere in the body following initial treatment, but a few do. If a breast cancer spreads, most commonly it metastasizes to the lungs and the bones. The idea was to look for early evidence of metastatic cancer in these areas, which could then be followed by early additional treatment.

Over 1,200 women with breast cancer were randomized into one of two groups: clinical follow-up (seeing their doctors in clinic and getting a mammogram) or intensive follow-up (the addition of other tests to examine the lungs and bones). So this intervention sought multiple pieces of information all directed at the same question: Has the cancer metastasized?

In one sense, the study worked. Women in the intensive follow-up group who developed metastatic cancer did have their lung and bone metastases found earlier. In another sense, it did not. The death rate, again, went in the wrong direction—it was slightly higher in the group with more information. That's three for three. But, again, all this could be the result of chance. From a statistical standpoint we would say there was no difference in death between the groups.

But from my standpoint—and the authors' and most oncologists'—the real effect was harm. Not because of the death rate, but because of the nature of the information. Women in the intensive follow-up group were told earlier that their cancer had spread. They were told earlier that their cancer was incurable. A similar trial added liver imaging into the mix and got a similar result.

Searching for evidence of metastatic cancer can be terrifying to cancer patients. My wife has a cadre of breast cancer buddies—women Linda befriended while they were all in treatment—and it was interesting to learn how differently they were treated, despite all being treated at the same institution. Ruth had a doctor who was always on the lookout for metastatic disease. New cough? Could be the cancer in the lungs. Better get a CT. Sore ankle? Could be the cancer in the bones. Better get an MRI. The fact that Ruth had just taken a positive step for her health—by picking up running again—apparently wasn't relevant. Reporting any discomfort produced a new scare—followed by a waiting period to get the test, and another to get the verdict. Stress without purpose. Ruth said she felt her doctor had "taken years off my life." I'm so glad Linda's oncologist was in a different place: thinking a new cough was more likely a cold—and a sore ankle was more likely a sprain—than a cancer metastasis.

Not to pile on, but an analogous study in colon cancer patients was just published as I was writing this. It investigated the utility of a blood test commonly used to detect the spread of colon cancer (carcinoembryonic antigen—aka CEA) along with CT scans of the chest, abdomen, and pelvis. And it had a similar result: more information led to more detection of metastases, more cancer surgery, and a statistically unchanged death rate—which was, yet again, slightly higher in the "more information" group.

That's four for four. What are the chances of that?

Seeking information about early signs of metastatic cancer doesn't help cancer patients live longer. But it does scare many and leads a few to live longer with the knowledge that they have incurable disease. They are subjected to additional therapies and their toxicities earlier—at a time when they would be otherwise asymptomatic.

Sometimes shining the light doesn't help, it hurts.

DATA VERSUS USEFUL KNOWLEDGE

While I like science, I'm not a big fan of semantics. But I have learned that words matter. And by now you may be wondering whether *information* is the right word. Information has the connotation of something that is always useful. As the foregoing trials suggest, however, it's not always useful. And if there's no advantage to knowing your cancer has come back—knowing this fact earlier as opposed to later sure sounds like something less than useful, more like harmful. A more precise vocabulary is needed.

One approach is to distinguish data from information—and information from useful knowledge. I first learned of these distinctions in 1990 when I read a *Washington Post* article by Ken Ringle on the opening of the "Information Age" exhibit at the Smithsonian Institution. The information age begins with the dawn of computing—which in turn is an outgrowth of World War II. The war effort had scientists working with reams of data, not only as part of the Manhattan Project to develop the atomic bomb, but also as part of the effort to unmask intercepted radio traffic of Nazi Germany and Japan. The radio traffic was encoded using a cipher machine called—appropriately enough—an enigma. Primitive computers ultimately unmasked the enigma-ciphered radio traffic. And the display of the process led Mr. Ringle to identify the limitation of the "Information Age" exhibit—not to mention the limitation of the age itself.

> Fascinating as the code-breaking section of "Information Age" is, however, it is there that the limitations of the exhibit begin to become apparent. What better spot to underline the differences between **data** (enciphered radio traffic itself), **information** (what it meant when decoded) and **useful knowledge** (what that told us about the enemy's intentions), not to mention **wisdom** (what strategy to follow as a result)?

Data, information, useful knowledge, wisdom . . . that's a good vocabulary. Good enough for me to keep the article around for a quarter century. I might tweak the definitions a bit for clinical medicine. Data would be the measurements of lung impedance. They would only become information if they reliably told us about the likelihood that the patient would develop a clinical problem (shortness of breath)—a problem that might lead to a hospitalization. The information would become useful knowledge only if we had a course of action that reliably lowered that likelihood. Wisdom requires balancing the benefits and harms of that action—and knowing how the patient values the various outcomes—to arrive at a decision about what to do.

Just because you have data doesn't mean you have information. Having information doesn't mean you have useful knowledge. And wisdom—well, that's a whole new ball game.

Mr. Ringle argued the Smithsonian exhibit failed to make these distinctions, overwhelmed the visitor with data overload, and would have benefited from more selectivity. More importantly, he made the same critique of the information age itself—that the increasing ease of storing and retrieving data *("What the hell, let's file it all")* has eliminated the need for the sort of value judgments about what is important. It is too easy to drown in data.

> The results bombard us daily from our newspapers, radios and television sets and account in no small part for the anxiety that imbues our time.

Wow. And that was written before the advent of full-body scanning, personal genetic testing, and smartphone biometric monitoring.

The central question for this chapter is whether obtaining more clinical data on individuals with medical problems reliably leads to useful knowledge. The short answer is: no. The natural follow-up question is whether there is any reason—other than cost—not to obtain more clinical data. The short answer is: yes. More clinical data not only can create anxiety for patients, they can also initiate cascades that lead to unneeded medical care.

The problem is twofold. First, there are clinical data that provide real information (such as detecting a breast cancer metastasis) but not useful knowledge. They have no utility in terms of therapy, yet have real disutility in terms of the patient's sense of well-being and resilience—components of the state of mind that is central to our health. Second, there are clinical data that do not provide genuine information—much less useful knowledge—since there is just too little signal and too much noise (such as measuring electrical impedance in the lung). These data simply produce too many alarms—alarms that we doctors tend to feel we have to react to—and that can distract us from what's important.

And if there are reasons not to seek more clinical data in patients who already have a medical problem, you might imagine there are reasons not to seek more clinical data in people who are well.

BRUCE'S BIG HEART

I ran into Bruce totally unexpectedly in Montana (he lives in Alaska; I live in Vermont). I had first met him a decade earlier at a meeting. He is about my age and he is also a physician. That's where our similarities end. I'm a primary care practitioner; Bruce is an intensivist. That's not a personality disorder, it's a medical specialty. Intensivists are the doctors who work in intensive care units, the part of the hospital where we send the most acutely ill patients. These patients often have multiple organs that are in trouble—kidney problems, heart problems, lung problems, and brain problems. They are the sickest of the sick.

Intensivists monitor these patients continually, with the help of multiple technologies that literally have bells and whistles that alert them to changing conditions. There are lots of tubes, wires, and data displays showing heart rate, heart tracings, blood pressure, respiratory rate, oxygen levels, and urinary output. Intensivists respond to those changes by changing fluid administration, intravenous drug therapy, and ventilator settings. The doctors quickly get feedback on their actions displayed on the various monitors. If a monitor shows a fast heart rate, we respond by administering a drug to slow it, and a few minutes later the monitor looks different. Problem solved. I loved this kind of work as a trainee—I used to feel like I was on the bridge of the starship *Enterprise*—but I don't think I'd have the stamina for it now (my wife says I should change "stamina" to "stomach," but that's a different story).

My point is: Bruce knows sick patients—and he understands how to deal with a lot of data. But he also understands how too much data can be a problem. In fact, he wishes he didn't understand the problem so well from personal experience.

When he turned fifty he decided to be screened for colon cancer. He went to his primary care practitioner, who was happy to set that up but also wanted to do a bunch of other tests. Bruce was hesitant, understanding that more data can be a two-edged sword. He said no to a chest X-ray; he said no to a cholesterol check.

His doctor said, "Let me at least get an EKG." An EKG is a simple test. Twelve pads are attached to the chest and extremities, and a few seconds later there is a printed page showing the electrical activity of the heart. It's a great test for patients having chest pain or for patients having trouble maintaining their blood pressure. Bruce looks at them every day in the intensive care unit.

Bruce was still hesitant, but knew the chances were very good that he would have a normal EKG. He felt well. He had no heart disease in his family. More importantly, he knew he was fit. He enjoyed exercising vigorously—and he could do so without any problems (he rode a bike more than a hundred miles per week until the snow fell; then it was time for Nordic skiing). He wasn't worried about heart disease; he was worried about being labeled as being a "difficult patient." So he accepted the test.

He wishes he hadn't. His EKG was wildly abnormal. It suggested that the wall of Bruce's heart was very thick. Too thick. The next step is to get an image of the heart to look at its anatomy. He got an echocardiogram (an ultrasound of the heart) and it was also abnormal. Bruce asked a cardiologist friend what he should do; he suggested a cardiac MRI.

Getting a high-quality MRI image of a beating heart is way more technically challenging than getting an EKG. It requires more than simply buying an expensive machine. There are many decisions to make: how to choose the imaging plane, how to synchronize the imaging with the heartbeat, and how to balance the trade-off between temporal resolution, spatial resolution, and imaging time. And once you have a high-quality image there is still the whole question of interpretation: you still need someone who knows what they are looking at.

So Bruce wanted to go somewhere where a lot of cardiac MRIs were done. He went to Rochester, Minnesota, home of the Mayo Clinic.

Mayo has cardiologists who look at MRIs every day and have cardiology subspecialists who just treat patients with thick hearts—that's all they do. He figured it would be the best place to go for an opinion about what he should do.

Bruce has nothing but good to say about Mayo. As an Alaskan physician, he gives them high marks for their phone consultation provided to doctors outside the system who are treating patients with unusual problems. As a patient, he was impressed with how kind, how personable, how knowledgeable, and how efficient their employees were at every step of his care. They did the MRI—plus blood work, plus the EKG again, plus the echocardiogram again, plus overnight oxygen monitoring, plus overnight heart rhythm monitoring. An exercise physiologist took sophisticated measurements of his heart and lung function while he exercised vigorously on a bicycle. Based on these measurements, it was clear Bruce could exercise much better than most people his age. His heart had been stressed and it passed with flying colors.

The cardiologist sat down with him to convey the final diagnosis: nonobstructive hypertrophic cardiomyopathy.

"What should I do?" Bruce asked.

"Come back and see us in three years," the cardiologist said.

That wasn't a very satisfying answer. But it was probably the right one. At least it was the consensus answer from the American College of Cardiology and the American Heart Association in 2011. Here is their guideline for asymptomatic patients with hypertrophic cardiomyopathy:

> It is recommended that comorbidities that may contribute to cardiovascular disease (e.g., hypertension, diabetes, hyperlipidemia, obesity) be treated in compliance with relevant existing guidelines.

In other words, the only treatments suggested are those that a doctor would suggest for a patient without hypertrophic cardiomyopathy.

The diagnosis was not helpful. There was nothing for Bruce to do, except worry.

Most affected individuals probably achieve a normal life expectancy without disability or the necessity for major therapeutic interventions. On the other hand, in some patients, hypertrophic cardiomyopathy is associated with disease complications that may be profound, with the potential to result in disease progression or premature death.

The phrase "premature death" is meant to refer to sudden cardiac death—the kind of death that happens out of the blue. Bruce worried that he might become hypersensitive about any sensation coming from his chest while biking or skiing. Is that heartburn? A muscle twinge? Or cardiac pain? Exercise that he really enjoyed might not be so enjoyable anymore.

Oh, the Mayo cardiologist did have one suggestion: genetic testing. What would be the rationale for genetic testing? It turns out hypertrophic cardiomyopathy is typically a genetic disorder involving one of more than 1,400 mutations among at least 8 genes. So Bruce could be tested for some of the more common mutations. If he tested positive, then he could worry more, both about himself and his four children. They could be tested. If any of the kids tested positive, then they could worry too—along with Bruce and his wife.

Bruce wasn't signing up for that deal. He stopped this train. Too much scary data; no useful knowledge.

DATA DREDGING IN THE WELL: GENETIC TESTING AND HOME MONITORING

We are entering a world where you can obtain lots of biometric data about yourself. You can already test various portions of your genome; there is little doubt you will soon be able to readily sequence the whole thing. You can already have your blood pressure, oxygen saturation, and blood sugar monitored by mobile devices; there is little doubt you will soon be able to monitor multiple physiological and biochemical variables on your smartphone—or on your new smartwatch.

What drives this? Two things. First, economics—the potential market is huge. Those engaged in the business of testing don't want to be confined to the relatively few sick patients; they want to test everybody. Second, the assumption that it never hurts to get more information— or, more precisely, it never hurts to get more data.

Some see these developments as transforming medicine, empowering patients with data, and engaging them in their own health care. United HealthCare has an advertising campaign featuring satisfied customers with a sea of numbers swirling around them accompanied by the slogan "Health in Numbers."

I'm less sanguine. I see unselected biometric data as producing the same problems as screening—leading people to feel more vulnerable, to be terrorized by false alarms, and to be overdiagnosed and overtreated. Only here, these problems are on steroids. At least screening is focused on the early diagnosis of a specific disease; collecting a sea of unselected numbers, pixels, and sequences feels more like a fishing expedition. And don't think light-footprint fly fishing here, think bottom trawling—dragging a net across the ocean floor and catching just about everything. It's data dredging.

"What the hell, let's file it all."

The need for selectivity in this setting is huge. We shouldn't be driven by what's possible; we should be driven by what's useful. Data obtained via genetic testing and home monitoring must be distinguished from useful knowledge.

Of course, genetic testing can be useful. There are a few genetic abnormalities that represent genuine information—such as the mutations associated with Huntington's disease, cystic fibrosis, and breast and ovarian cancer. They provide genuine information because these gene mutations are so reliably associated with clinical disease (the geneticists would say that since the genotype is closely linked to the phenotype, these mutations are highly penetrant).

But even here there is a choice to be made. Why? Because for some, the information is not useful knowledge. Some people choose not to know they are destined to develop the degenerative neurologic disorder of Huntington's disease, because there's nothing to be done about it. Some couples choose not to know whether their unborn child is destined to have cystic fibrosis, because they would not consider ending the pregnancy. And some women choose not to know whether they have one of the so-called BRCA mutations (although BRCA stands for *BReast CAncer*, the mutations are strongly associated with both breast and ovarian cancer). In response to a commentary I wrote following Angelina Jolie's decision to be tested (and prophylactically treated, because she had a BRCA mutation), one wrote explaining her thinking:

> You might be wondering right now if I've been tested for BRCA2. Surely only a crazy person would choose not to get this test when a family member died due to complications of this gene mutation, right? The answer is, for now, I have chosen not to get tested.
>
> Why? Because I don't want to know. Not right now. I'm 27 years old. I don't want to be burdened with the knowledge that I have a gene mutation. I don't want to be rushed into having kids so I can have a double mastectomy and a complete hysterectomy by 30 "just in case."
>
> I'm not going to be pressured into extreme decisions just because a celebrity made them. No one should. Yes, knowledge is power, but ignorance is bliss.

At least genetic testing is a one-time deal; home monitoring is repetitive testing. Of course, home monitoring can be useful. Home glucose monitoring is an important tool for patients taking drugs to lower their blood sugar, particularly insulin. Home blood pressure monitoring provides much needed additional readings of patients' blood pressure when they are not in the doctor's office—where blood pressure is frequently spuriously high. Like most primary care physicians, I have patients using both technologies. And, truth be told, I have monitored my own blood pressure at home off and on over the past decade.

But, again, selectivity is called for. There are way too many patients monitoring their glucose at home. The information is not that useful—although it is a great business, particularly the test strips (the United

Kingdom's National Health Service reported that more was spent on test strips than the oral medications to lower blood sugar). While patients are carefully recording their blood sugar (often multiple times a day), physicians are increasingly basing their management decisions on hemoglobin A1c, a lab test that measures average blood sugar over time. The real reason to monitor glucose is to make sure it doesn't go too low, and that would be less of a problem if doctors weren't so aggressive in lowering blood sugar—which we now know can be harmful.

The case is stronger for blood pressure monitoring, but both monitoring efforts share a similar drawback: patients may place undue emphasis on a single high reading. Both blood pressure and blood sugar vary considerably across the day. If patients happen to catch a high value, it leads them to worry—or feel that they are somehow not doing things right. For patients with type 2 diabetes (again, that's the most common type of diabetes—the type that typically occurs in obese adults) who are not using insulin (that's most of them), investigators in Italy's nationwide initiative for diabetes quality found that home glucose monitoring led to more distress and depression, particularly if patients ran tests more than once a day. And more frequent home monitoring didn't help patients better manage their disease.

The ability to make biometric measurements has led to grandiose visions for how more biometric data will keep us well. Over a decade ago, the ability to sequence genes led to the vision of a baseline genome scan: all young adults would be tested to determine their risk for various diseases. What happened to that vision? There were loads of data but not much useful knowledge. Genes are only one determinant of your health, and very few are reliably predictive of any one disease. Finding lots of weak relationships—for which it is not clear anything different should be done—is not useful. Nor is finding lots and lots of what the geneticists call "variants of uncertain significance"—it's the genetic version of noise.

That's why, in 2013, the FDA brought the hammer down on 23andme. It is one of several commercial enterprises promoting genetic testing to individuals (the 23 refers to the number of chromosomal pairs in the human genome). The company has a strong data lineage—it is backed by Google and run by the wife of a Google cofounder—and had been telling people they had genetic profiles that predisposed them to specific diseases. But whether the genomic data provide accurate information, much less useful knowledge, remains unclear. FDA has had a long-standing mandate to protect us from snake oil treatments; now they are recognizing that protecting us from snake oil testing is every bit as important.

So we move on. Genes are static; to stay well, we're now being told you need to be regularly monitored. There is a developing mobile-health industry, or m-health, producing devices and apps to "give people dashboards, gauges and alarm signals" (according to a representative of Qualcomm Life). The dashboards can already include gauges for temperature, heart rate, respiratory rate, blood pressure, blood sugar, and oxygen saturation, as well as EKGs. That's a lot of gauges to monitor— and a lot of potential alarms.

M-health is sold on a double promise: (1) it will make the population healthier and (2) it will save money by alerting people to action before they need expensive treatment. But it is equally plausible that m-health will do just the reverse: (1) it will make the population feel more vulnerable and less healthy and (2) it will cost money—both for the equipment and because people have to seek medical care to get their alarms turned off.

And fancier monitoring gauges are coming down the pike, including this one from HealthTell:

> The challenge right now in diagnostics, when you go to see the doctor, is by the time you catch a lot of diseases it's often too late. So, for example, for cancer you have to see it—on an X-ray, CT scan, or a scope. And so the ideal, of course, is to be able to take something less invasive—like a little bit of blood or a sputum sample—and to be able to detect that much earlier. . . . Our vision of the future is that instead of having to go to the doctor, and having to get reimbursed for a $2,000 test, you can actually mail in a drop of blood or a swab in an envelope and we would—on a continual basis—monitor your health.

Send me a drop of your blood every month. That's the vision of the CEO of HealthTell, one of the start-ups focusing on molecular diagnosis—measuring the activity of your own immune system (the so-called immunosignature)—to test for various diseases, such as Alzheimer's disease, HIV, and cancer. It's a vision in which the well could be continually monitored for an expanding number of diseases.

Is this snake oil? It's certainly a reasonable question to ask. No one knows how well immunosignatures predict disease. In fact, the worst diseases may well be those that don't produce any immune response—that have no immunosignature.

And the question of what people who otherwise feel well should do if their immunosignature is deemed to be "concerning" remains totally unanswered. At least they can worry.

I don't want to stifle innovation, but wouldn't it be nice if this kind of energy and vision was directed to those who had problems, instead of to finding (and creating) new problems for those who do not?

EASY TO COLLECT DATA; HARD TO PRODUCE USEFUL KNOWLEDGE

I remember sharing the problem of too much data with a group of medical students. One of them asked, "Isn't the real problem not the data but the parameterization?" To which my response was "Huh?" Turns out he is part of an increasingly common—and, from my standpoint, desirable—trend in medical education: students who train in medicine after having had another career. He was an engineer.

I think I now know what he was asking. We know, for example, that cloud formation is a function of two variables: temperature and humidity. But temperature is a function of how much solar radiation hits the ground and how much heat is radiated back into space. That, in turn, is affected by clouds. Without even considering the determinants of humidity—or the fact that air moves around—all of a sudden there are a lot of moving pieces. We know the relevant variables, but we can't predict how they interact or affect one another. That's a parameterization problem.

And if we are challenged in parameterizing dynamic physical processes, you might imagine things could get really tough with dynamic biological processes.

Consider our evolving understanding of the single most important biometric measurement in human health. What's my nomination for the single most important biometric variable? Blood pressure. Not temperature, not heart rate, not respiratory rate, not oxygen saturation, not blood sugar, and not urine output (despite my being a big fan of that variable). And certainly not your immunosignature . . .

Some might point out that I'm cheating, because blood pressure is really two variables—a top and a bottom number. The top number is the highest pressure (when the heart contracts); the bottom number is the lowest pressure (immediately prior to the contraction). Two variables in one pick, that's not fair. Gotta pick one.

That's easy, I'll take the top number: systolic blood pressure.

That sure as hell isn't what I was taught in medical school. When I was in medical school (this is the point when my class of medical students yawns in unison), the focus was completely on the bottom number—diastolic blood pressure. It's like we didn't even know the top number existed. That is because all the early studies showing the benefit of treating very high blood pressure focused on the lower number. The first publication of the findings of the VA Cooperative Study of Hypertension, for example, enrolled men based on their diastolic blood pressures: 115 to 129 mmHg. That's really high. And the tremendous amount of benefit—within one year, 26 percent experienced a cardiovascular event in the untreated group versus less than 2 percent in the treated group—remains the standard against which all preventive interventions should be judged.

But in the ensuing years there has been a growing recognition that systolic is where the genuine information is, particularly as people age and cardiovascular events become more common. Isolated systolic hypertension (high systolic, normal diastolic) is clearly a problem. But it is less clear that isolated diastolic hypertension is a problem.

None of this invalidates the findings of the VA study in any way. It turned out to be a study of systolic hypertension—the average systolic pressure of enrolled patients was really high as well: 180 mmHg.

Medicine's shifting focus from diastolic to systolic blood pressure is a remarkable course correction—damn near a 180-degree turn. How could we be focused on the wrong variable for decades? One explanation is intellectual inertia: when we commit to one school of thought, it takes time to move to another. But it also takes time to do the research that overturns the prevailing mindset.

And there is an emerging, controversial school of thought that the genuine information might actually be in the pulse pressure—the difference between the systolic and diastolic blood pressure. If high pulse pressures become the prevailing explanatory variable for how high blood pressure adversely affects human health, high diastolic pressures might actually become good . . .

OK, maybe we do have parameterization problems. All of a sudden cholesterol is not as important as it used to be. Neither is "strict" control of blood sugar. These are biometric data that have also been around for decades, and we are still trying to decide under what conditions they provide useful knowledge. And these are relatively simple variables—there are two measures of blood pressure, two primary fractions of cholesterol, and two measures of blood sugar. There are thousands of genetic variants; there will be thousands of immunosignatures.

I'm all for more data on what the data mean. We have studied, and we will continue to study, how biometric variables are related to human health. The exponential improvement in computing power may help us evaluate this question faster. Then again, computational time is not what holds up the evaluation.

Two other elements require time. The first is collecting the data. While we are increasingly able to amass biometric data quickly, it takes time to observe the outcomes we care about: death, heart attack, and cancer. It takes even more time to determine whether actions taken based on biometric findings actually help people live longer or better. Nowhere is this more true than in studying the value of actions in those who are well, which can require studying thousands of individuals who are followed for decades.

The second is conceptualizing the problem. The initial conceptualization of high blood pressure happened to focus on the wrong variable; the course correction took years. Relationships that seem certain on initial inspection may be much less certain when inspected more carefully. Simplifying assumptions—like a linear relationship between exposure and outcome—can be horribly wrong. Course corrections are the norm; they take time.

Figuring out how to monitor something is a lot easier than figuring out what the data obtained from monitoring mean.

ANNUAL PHYSICALS: CHECKUP OR CHECK-IN?

Considering the utility of unselected data gathering leads to one of the most fundamental questions of medicine: What is the role of the annual physical?

First a little background: there's not a lot of science on the usefulness of the annual physical—and what science there is suggests it doesn't help people. Furthermore, the term "annual physical" is too narrow. It implies a yearly physical exam—looking into your eyes and ears, listening to your heart and lungs, palpating your abdomen, topped off with a rectal exam. Strictly speaking, all this could be done without talking to you. So a more accurate term is regular checkup or routine visit.

Whatever you call it, this is a big piece of primary care. Particularly for helping older patients age well—the setting for which I'd argue the case for regular checkups is strongest. I'm a primary care practitioner, so I've done a lot of them. I'm not professing expertise here; I'm disclosing potential bias.

There are different visions for what might take place during a regular checkup. One is an exhaustive search to see if we can find something wrong with you, something that you did not know about. It's the approach many of us were taught in medical school—a full court press to gather data: a structured interview regarding your bodily functions (we call it a review of systems), followed by a complete head-to-toe physical, followed by a series of tests. Because all of us harbor abnormalities, this kind of checkup can literally make you sick.

This approach can feel very isolating—physicians focused on your physical attributes, not on how you are feeling. Many primary care practitioners have altered the approach to regular checkups based on what they learned from their patients. I am no exception.

I learned something about what an aging population needs from another long-standing patient of mine, Mr. Roberts. I also learned from a mistake: I played a big role in breaking his neck.

At age seventy-four, Mr. Roberts was found to have an elevated blood sugar by routine testing. Subsequent testing confirmed the diagnosis: type 2 diabetes. He needed a primary care doctor; I was the new guy with available slots in my clinic. I started him on a medication to lower his blood sugar. And the medication worked well at lowering his blood sugar.

Six months later he blacked out while driving on the local interstate highway. His car went off the road and rolled over. His neck was broken in two places: he had fractured both his sixth and seventh cervical vertebrae. The paramedics on the scene measured his blood sugar. It was extremely low. The medication had worked *too* well.

As you might imagine, a broken neck encouraged me to think a little more about U-shaped curves. I'm not sure what happened. I had used the standard starting dose of medication. He had tolerated it without problems for almost half a year. Maybe he hadn't eaten normally that day; maybe he had a stomach bug. I don't know. But I do know the drug ultimately caused the accident—and that I had started the drug.

Because I saw him over the next fifteen years, I also know something else: he didn't need the drug in the first place. I never tried to treat his diabetes again and he never developed symptoms or complications from the disease. Treating him was a mistake.

I got to know Mr. Roberts well. He was born at the end of World War I and grew up in the mill towns built along the tributaries of the Connecticut River. These tributaries arise in the Vermont and New

Hampshire highlands on both sides of the Connecticut—the river is the state line—and are big enough to power all sorts of mills: textiles to machine tools. They are also big enough to flood badly, as they did on the Vermont side in 2011 during Hurricane Irene. As a kid, Mr. Roberts worked in the mills. As a young man he fought in World War II. He returned and found a job as a caretaker for a large piece of property. He married, had two children, and lost his wife a decade later.

He had some medical problems that I didn't cause. He had a portion of his colon missing—it had been surgically removed to treat inflammatory bowel disease years earlier. Consequently, he had a lot of diarrhea. But he and I figured out how to manage that. He became short of breath and developed pneumonia. Antibiotics fixed that. His heart beat too fast and he became light-headed. Cardiac medications managed that. He had bloody stools and became anemic. I could never figure out where the blood was coming from—neither could my colleagues in gastroenterology—but iron fixed the problem. Mr. Roberts had multiple medical problems.

And what did we talk about virtually every visit? Boston sports.

Hey, who knew that knowing something about Boston professional sports teams might be relevant to patient care in northern New England? For those who hate the Boston sports teams—notably the Boston Red Sox and the New England Patriots—I say fine; a lot of my high school buddies in Colorado would be in your camp. But understand, these were his local teams and their performance mattered to him. The *Boston Globe* circulates throughout northern New England. Mr. Roberts grew up listening to baseball on the radio. He knew the voice of the Red Sox was Curt Gowdy, and he heard him call the games regularly after the war (although I don't think he knew Curt was from western Wyoming). He was a running back throughout high school, at a time when soft leather was considered head protection. As he got older and moved into assisted living, his major purchase was a big-screen TV. Of course, he was a serious Boston sports fan.

For those of you who hate professional sports in general—the competitiveness, the focus on money—I apologize for the distraction. And for those of you who think that if the NFL wants to engage in health promotion, it might be more appropriate to focus on head injury (or domestic violence) than "the crucial catch" for breast cancer screening—I totally agree.

It's not just sports. Some of my patients want to talk about fishing or hunting. Others want to talk about new markets for dairy products or what's happening on their woodlot. Some want to talk about the weather; others want to talk politics—particularly New Hampshire veterans during primary season. It's easy to deride such small talk in medical care as being unimportant, even wasteful. But it's not all about data collection; connecting with people is a central part of primary care—central to the "caring" function of medicine. I got to know Mr. Roberts, and as he got older I got to know his daughters. He looked forward to seeing me; I looked forward to seeing him. We both knew he was reaching the end of life, and I knew how he wanted to approach that transition. I could assist with small things, prevent excessive medical care, and help him die at home.

So here is a different vision for the annual visit: less of a checkup, more of a check-in. This vision requires that the doctor focuses on actually talking with you, learning about what, if anything, is bothering you and what is going on with your life: your marriage, your children, your job, and your parents. This discussion, along with a few simple tests (such as for weight or blood pressure) and a little family history, gives your doctor a sense of what health risks you face. Then the doctor can present your options for minimizing those risks. The focus is on learning about you and promoting your health in a way that fits your approach to life. The check-in should be a conversation, not a concerted effort to look for things that are wrong.

DOWNSIDES OF MORE DATA

While assumptions about the value of clinical information are widespread, there is less understanding of the downsides of more data. To be sure, everybody understands the cost issue: laboratory testing, medical scanning, genetic sequencing, and biometric monitoring all cost money. And all too often, we're talking real money—thousands of dollars. But even if we had all the money in the world, there are reasons not to routinely seek more data. Let me summarize them here.

Distraction: Sometimes focusing on small things distracts us from seeing big things. Minor laboratory abnormalities identified during a routine visit (slightly elevated cholesterol level, slightly depressed thyroid function), for example, often draw both physicians and their patients away from problems more relevant to health (stopping smoking, getting more exercise, improving diet). Doctors like these distractions because they are more "actionable"; patients like them because the actions required are minimal—taking a pill. While the opportunities for distraction grow as more testing occurs, the resulting actions are not likely to make patients feel better.

For the sick, having their physicians distracted from their central problem is yet more concerning. Again, the opportunities for physicians to be overwhelmed with data are continually increasing. The problem is exemplified in the increasing ability to characterize the genetics of various cancers. We used to focus on a few tumor genes; now some are sequencing the entire tumor genome. And we are now recognizing that some cancers have multiple clones—in other words, different cells within the tumor have different genomes. Complete DNA sequencing of multiple genomes represents millions of data points. One oncologist characterized the resulting challenge as "drinking from a fire hose."

Radiologists know the problem as they have faced the issue in the increasing resolution of images—more data per cubic centimeter. A patient with intermittent abdominal pain was referred to me after being seen in the ER twenty-four hours earlier. He had had an abdominal CT scan and the radiology reading had identified multiple small abnormalities—nodules in the liver, kidney, and adrenal gland—none of which had anything to do with his pain. I went to the radiology department to have my "go to" radiologist review the study. First he wanted to hear the history, then he had the computer reconstruct the CT so that it appeared like a plain X-ray of the abdomen—the test that would have been done prior to the advent of CT.

It showed the source of the symptoms nicely: a loop of colon was caught between the diaphragm and the liver (it even has a name: Chilaiditi syndrome). While the CT could have found a small colon cancer, it's harder for it to identify a colon out of position. It's a classic "can't see the forest for the trees" problem.

Of course, the distraction of having too much data is not unique to medicine. World War II bombers dropped chaff—a cloud of small strips of aluminum—as a way to produce data overload and distract radar-guided searchlights used by antiaircraft gunners. Psychologists have argued that offering consumers too many options can distract them from making a decision. Intelligence analysts are questioning the utility of mass surveillance in the prevention of terrorism because it produces so much distracting data.

Having more data is not a uniform good. When faced with the problem of searching for a needle in the haystack—throwing more hay on the pile only makes the needle harder to find. And for the well, typically there is no needle to find. For them, more data are just distracting.

Anxiety: More data often translates to more scares. There is something new to worry about. You were worried about your hoarseness, now you are worried about your kidney cancer. You weren't worried about anything, now you are worried about your heart. And I'll never forget what happened to my wife after she found a breast lump and got a diagnostic mammogram (note: while there is considerable debate about the value of screening mammograms, doctors agree that diagnostic mammograms are valuable to help sort out whether a new breast lump is worrisome). Linda was worried about breast cancer because her mammogram was categorized as class 5—one that is indicative of a 95 percent chance of breast cancer—and she came out of her surgical appointment worried about thyroid cancer as well.

OK. A brief digression on thyroid cancer might be useful here. Pathologists have known for years that the thyroid is full of turtles—at least one-third of adults harbor small papillary thyroid cancers. Now we are starting to find them: since the mid-1990s the incidence of thyroid cancer detection in the United States has increased threefold, while the death rate has remained stable. That doesn't sound like an epidemic of real disease; that sounds like an epidemic of diagnosis. And the United States doesn't get the gold medal on this one; South Korea does. Their death rate is stable too, yet they have had a fifteen-fold increase in thyroid cancer detection. Needless to say, overdiagnosis is a huge problem in thyroid cancer.

These population statistics can feel sterile—they are, after all, just numbers. But they are numbers that reflect real people. I just learned that a family friend, again about my age, was recently found to have a small papillary thyroid cancer (recall, that has the word "*turtle*" written all over it). He survived surgery but had a stroke. Not a massive stroke mind you—he has just lost sensation and function of his lower arm and lower leg and also has some problem enunciating his words. Intraoperative stroke is rare, but it is undoubtedly more common than anything bad happening had he left the small papillary thyroid cancer alone and waited to see if it became a problem. So again, just because it happens rarely doesn't mean that it doesn't happen.

So how is a woman worried about breast cancer (with good reason, given a class 5 mammogram) made to worry about thyroid cancer? Because her surgeon was collecting more data. He prided himself on examining all his patients for thyroid cancer—and he found a nodule in Linda's neck. Most of us could be found to have nodules in our neck, particularly if our doctors looked hard enough. Before he examined her breast, before he reviewed her mammogram—he was recommending a thyroid biopsy. I was dumbfounded; Linda wanted a new surgeon. (That was almost twenty years ago. If she has thyroid cancer, it's a turtle.)

It is tempting to downplay these emotional effects. Psychosocial issues seem so much less important than the "life-and-death" stuff. But many conditions that we think of as life-and-death issues turn out not to be. Data about them are not useful knowledge; they are distractions. But in the meantime the resiliency of patients gets worn down: they feel more fragile, more vulnerable. Health is not simply the absence of physical abnormality; it's also a state of mind. Having too much data undermines that state.

Cascade effect: The cascade effect may sound like physics—or maybe a better pick would be a fluvial process in geology. I should define the term. Better yet, I'll defer to Mold and Stein, who originally introduced the problem to physicians in 1986:

> The cascade effect that we will describe generally consists of an initiating factor or factors, followed by a series of events that seem to be a direct result of previous events, often catalyzed by some characteristic of the system—usually anxiety [that's not just patient anxiety, it's physician anxiety as well]. This chain of events tends to proceed with increasing momentum, so that the further it progresses, the more difficult it is to stop.

The initiating factor for a medical cascade is typically an extraneous data point. Mr. Baker got caught in a cascade precipitated by a chest X-ray at the beginning of this chapter. Worse was Mr. Nadeau's cascade precipitated by a checkup described in the introduction. Why do I say worse? At least Mr. Baker had a reason to enter the medical care system—he was hoarse. Mr. Nadeau was trying to stay well. Check for an aortic aneurysm, find something worrisome in the pancreas. Get a better look—more data—and find something worrisome in the liver. Get a biopsy—more data—and get bleeding and urinary retention. Not to mention a week in the hospital and a bill for $50,000.

PRESCRIPTION: BE WARY OF FISHING EXPEDITIONS; ASK HOW MORE DATA WILL CHANGE WHAT YOU WILL DO

The value of information is a central tenet of twenty-first-century culture. But the tenet conflates data with useful knowledge; your job is to recognize the distinction.

If you are sick and in the medical care system, your physician will generally be the person deciding which data to obtain. Because of their increasing understanding that data can be a double-edged sword, it is increasingly likely your physician will understand the value of prudent test-ordering. Sharing that you recognize the distinction between data and useful knowledge only makes prudent test-ordering more likely. If, however, you worry that you are being excessively tested, I suggest you ask your doctor two questions:

What are we looking for? With this question, you are trying to determine whether there is a succinct answer (a specific diagnosis) or whether you are going on a fishing expedition (looking for anything wrong). Trying to find—or exclude—a specific diagnosis may make perfect sense. But be wary of fishing expeditions; it's too easy to catch trash fish.

If we find what we are looking for, what will we do differently? This is the acid-test question: Will the data change what we do? This may take more involvement on your part. The doctor may lay out various courses of action, and you have to decide what you would agree to. The bottom line is this: if the data won't change what you will do, don't seek the data.

If you are well, you will have more and more opportunity to decide to collect data about yourself. But recognize that getting more data is not always in your interest. You will have to decide what constitutes useful information. It certainly doesn't make sense to get more data, if you don't know what the data mean—or have no clue about what to do next.

Finally, whether you are sick or well, be open to question whether data from our machines actually represent useful information. It's particularly important to be skeptical when a test identifies a thoroughly unexpected finding—something out of left field, something your doctor wasn't even looking for, a total surprise. Surprising findings are most commonly associated with advanced medical imaging (CT scans, MRI, and the like). And they are common enough that more and more doctors are preparing patients for them—prior to the test. *"I'm looking for X, but this test sees so much that I won't be surprised if it finds some other things that I'll recommend we not worry about."*

It's good preparation—and it's good advice. As our diagnostic technologies are increasingly able to detect minute perturbations in our anatomy, physiology, biochemistry, and genome, surprising findings may not be all that surprising.

ACTION IS ALWAYS BETTER THAN INACTION

Disturbing truth: Action is not reliably the "right" choice

SOMETIMES DOING NOTHING IS exactly the right thing to do.

The first four chapters have all been about doing something: attempting to lower risk, trying to fix problems, looking for early forms of disease, and seeking more information. In each case, I've suggested there are reasons not to do something. So admittedly, I've already presented some of the argument for inaction.

In this chapter, I want to explore why taking action is so compelling. And I want to move beyond epidemiology, heart disease, cancer, and informatics to consider the area of medicine in which our actions are most dramatic: surgery.

A PRESIDENT WHO NEEDED INACTION

The president had been shot. Multiple doctors promptly engaged in his care.

I'm not referring to President Reagan in 1981 or President Kennedy in 1963—instead, I'm referring to President Garfield in 1881. The president was about to board a train to attend his twenty-fifth reunion at Williams College when he was shot in the waiting room of Washington's Baltimore and Potomac Station. The wound was not lethal, but the subsequent actions taken by his doctors certainly were.

I first read this intriguing assessment in Candace Millard's book *Destiny of the Republic*. As I looked at the bibliography, one name stood out: Dr. Donald Trunkey. I wanted to go to the source.

When doctors reflect back on their training, certain individuals stand out. These are the clinicians, the professors, and the mentors who get fixed in our memories over the years. A few loom larger than life. They are the giants of medicine. From my perspective, Dr. Trunkey is one of those giants. As a medical student, I traveled two thousand miles west to do a clerkship on his service in 1981. I had seen him on television—when he was featured in an episode of *Lifeline*, a short-lived NBC series documenting the daily routines of some of the nation's most prominent physicians.

Dr. Trunkey is a trauma surgeon, one who specializes in the care of severely wounded patients. In the 1970s and '80s he was the "go-to surgeon" at the public hospital for the City and County of San Francisco, San Francisco General. All of the city's trauma patients go there. If you get badly hurt in San Francisco, you'll be shipped to the General. And that's a good thing, because that's where you'll get the best trauma care.

During Dr. Trunkey's tenure, San Francisco was quite a wild city: plenty of drugs and plenty of crime. He gained a wealth of experience with what he calls penetrating trauma—what most of us would call knife and gunshot wounds. So I knew he was the right guy to talk to about President Garfield's medical care.

President Garfield was shot in the back with a .44 caliber pistol, at a distance of about six feet. At the autopsy the bullet's path was evident: after entering the skin about four inches lateral to the spinal column, it went on to fracture two ribs, and then it crossed the midline by going through the body of first lumbar vertebra, before finally coming to rest just behind the tail of the pancreas. Remarkable were the vital structures it missed: the spinal cord, the abdominal aorta, the pancreas itself, and the adjacent spleen. And it was remarkable that the autopsy that produced this information didn't occur until more than two months after the shooting. Why? Because the president didn't die until more than two months after the shooting.

I tracked Dr. Trunkey down in Portland, Oregon, where he had moved to serve as the chairman of surgery at the Oregon Health Sciences University. Although he has since stepped down, he still operates—and he still takes trauma call. I asked Dr. Trunkey about Garfield's care. His assessment was blunt. "He was killed by a surgeon."

Don't make the mistake of thinking this was a snap judgment made by an arrogant surgeon. Dr. Trunkey is an academic physician, someone who has carefully studied organized trauma systems and did seminal work demonstrating their value in saving lives. More relevant to the topic at hand, he has also studied the medical and surgical care given to our four assassinated presidents.

After Garfield was shot, you can imagine there was great pressure on his doctors to do something. President Lincoln had been assassinated only sixteen years earlier. The general consensus among the multiple doctors involved in Garfield's care seems to have been this: the thing to do was to figure out where the bullet was. That involved exploring the wound.

How did surgeons explore wounds at that time? By sticking their fingers in them. In the first few days following the shooting, President Garfield had his wound explored multiple times—by multiple surgeons. Each exam introduced more bacteria into the wound. But the surgeon's fingers were far too short to find the bullet—it was probably about a foot from where it had penetrated the skin. So they tried probes: malleable metal wire instruments that—while unable to detect the bullet—were able to introduce bacteria more deeply into the wound.

Three weeks later President Garfield had a temperature of 104. He had developed a large abscess—a collection of pus reflecting an infected wound. In subsequent weeks he developed pus collections in various parts of his body: in the skin, in the parotid gland, in the liver, in the lung, and in the kidney. He lost nearly one hundred pounds. Here was an otherwise healthy man dying of disseminated infection—an infection that was disseminated by actions taken by his doctors. At his trial, the man who shot the president admitted to the shooting, but not the murder. He laid that at the foot of the doctors. As does Dr. Trunkey.

The irony is this: had Garfield not been the president but instead an average Joe, he would almost certainly have lived. There were numerous Civil War veterans who just a few years earlier had survived bullet wounds of similar severity. What was done for them? Nothing. The bullet was allowed to stay where it was and the wound was allowed to heal.

INFECTION—ONE UNINTENDED CONSEQUENCE OF ACTION

Whenever there is a problem—even if it is less dramatic than a president being shot—there is a strong undercurrent to do something. There is an assumption that action is preferable to inaction—with the rationale typically expressed using the maxim "better safe than sorry." But in medical care the reality is that our actions have unintended consequences. As exemplified by the story of President Garfield's medical care, one unintended consequence of surgical intervention is infection. How doctors learned this is a classic story in medical history. But infection is not a problem that can be relegated to the past.

Some things are so evident with careful observation that randomized trials are not needed (as in, when jumping out of an airplane, parachutes are useful). Based on the observations of a Hungarian obstetrician—Ignaz Semmelweis—the utility of hand washing prior to surgery falls in that category.

The problem was puerperal fever: an infection, typically involving the uterus, in a female following childbirth. It became a very common problem in the nineteenth century, as the process of birth became medicalized and women in labor were housed in what were known as "lying-in" hospitals—where they were repeatedly checked by introducing hands (and instruments) into the vagina. Maternal mortality rates skyrocketed—as many as one-quarter of all new mothers died from puerperal fever.

Semmelweis's observations were made possible because he was responsible for, not one, but two birthing wards—and because he bothered to count the death rate from puerperal fever in each. One ward had the standard death rate for the time; the other a rate one-third of that. The two wards admitted women on alternate days—that's close to randomization—so Semmelweis knew that the difference was not because the women were different. What was different was this: one ward was the teaching service for medical students, while the other was for the instruction of midwives only.

You get to guess which was which. I'll give you a hint: the story doesn't end well for the doctors . . .

Turns out the medical students, in addition to providing obstetrical care, were also performing autopsies. It's the way we learn human anatomy as well as the way we learn why people die. And on whom were the medical students performing autopsies? The women who died from puerperal fever. They then walked a few feet and "assisted" women who were alive in their labor and delivery—without washing their hands.

That can't be good.

Lest you think I'm mocking the doctors of the time, I should be clear that they had no knowledge of germs—or, specifically, bacteria. But Semmelweis deduced what was happening. Although he didn't get the mechanism quite right (he concluded that some "cadaverous material" caused the puerperal fever), he sure got the solution right: wash your hands. Having the medical students wash their hands with a chlorinated solution between the autopsy and maternity suite led to a precipitous drop in the death rate from puerperal fever.

That was in 1847. In the early 1860s Louis Pasteur established the correct mechanism for the fever—microorganisms—and the germ theory of disease was born. A few years later a British surgeon, Joseph Lister, established the value of antiseptic techniques: having surgeons wear clean gloves, use clean instruments, and wash their hands.

Garfield was shot in 1881. Did I mention that course corrections in medicine take time?

In our discussions Dr. Trunkey was clear that American surgeons were aware of Lister's work. But they chose not to believe it. As late as the 1882 meeting of the American Surgical Association, the *Lancet* reported that "anti-Listerians were in the majority." You can bet that Garfield was not the only casualty of this belief.

INFECTION—IT'S NOT JUST ABOUT HAND WASHING

All surgeons now recognize that inserting nonsterile fingers into wounds is the wrong thing to do. It's useful knowledge. But the problem of surgical infection remains.

One of the worst complications emanating from medical care I provided was a surgical infection. In the early 1980s I was one of two surgical officers in the US Public Health Service Hospital in Bethel, Alaska. I had a very limited repertoire, largely confined to stabilizing major trauma prior to air evacuation, and doing two common (and relatively simple) operations: tubal ligation and appendectomy.

One of those appendectomies involved a man just my age (we were about thirty). Ed's operation went well, and there was nothing particularly noteworthy about it. I gave him antibiotics. But three days later the site of my incision started to produce pus. I called the surgeons in Anchorage to seek their advice. They had me take Ed back to the OR, remove the skin sutures, and reopen the wound so that it could drain. I packed the wound with sterile gauze and repacked it every day. The wound ultimately closed from the bottom up. He recovered fully but that process took time—as in three to four weeks. Ed and I developed a close relationship over those weeks, but I still felt bad about what had happened.

I had worn gloves. I had used sterilized instruments. I had washed my hands. I was not an anti-Listerian. Yet my patient had nonetheless developed a nasty wound infection.

The germ theory of disease gave bacteria a bad name. Now we are in the midst of a serious reassessment. We all harbor bacteria—a lot of them. The human body has many more bacteria than cells. In the digestive tract they serve as subcontractors: freestanding metabolic factories performing a variety of chemical reactions that are important to our digestion and nutrition, from breaking down complex carbohydrates to synthesizing vitamins. And there is emerging evidence that bacteria in the gut—and on the skin—help protect the body from infection.

So while some bacteria deserve a bad name, we now recognize that many are good for us. But it's definitely not good to have even good bacteria in the wrong place. Making an incision through the skin or the gut—both of which I did during Ed's appendectomy—is one way to get bacteria in the wrong place. Surgeons strive to avoid introducing their own bacteria into the incisions they make into patients. But infections of their incisions—so-called surgical site infections—are still a problem. Where do the bacteria come from? Typically they come from the patients themselves. It's not because patients are dirty; it's because we all harbor bacteria.

And the problem is bigger than just surgery. Medical care in general has a problem with infection. There is now a large literature on hospital-acquired infection, in which patients get infected as a consequence of their hospitalization. Why does this happen? A lot of attention is given to inadequate hygienic practices—particularly hand washing. While surgeons routinely wash their hands before surgery (and wear gloves), adherence to hand washing recommendations elsewhere in the hospital is typically below 50 percent.

But the problem of hospital-acquired infection isn't that simple (I'm tempted to say the hygiene folks have overplayed their hand). The bigger issue is this: hospitals, and other health-care institutions, are the settings in which things are done to people—things that weaken the body's defenses and increase the chance of infection. Medications are administered that have the side effect of compromising the immune system. Procedures are performed that disrupt the skin—the organ that serves as the protective layer of the body. Tubes are inserted, providing bacteria an easy path to the wrong place—serving as a portal of entry to the blood or the lungs. And antibiotics end up killing good bacteria, opening up a new ecological niche for the bad (antibiotic-associated diarrhea being the most familiar example).

The Centers for Disease Control has even broadened the concept of hospital-acquired infection to encompass all of medical care: using the term "health care–associated infections." They concluded that there were 1.7 million health care–associated infections in the United States during 2002—and they estimated these infections were associated with 98,987 deaths.

I don't know if that's the right number. I do know that juxtaposing the number "98,987" with the word "estimate" is laughable. Shouldn't the estimate be "about 100,000"? And many of these deaths could also be associated with (pick one) obesity, diabetes, vascular disease, or cigarette smoking. So there's more than a little double counting going on here.

I apologize. That drew a flag from the refs—unnecessary roughness. I should have just said: I don't know if that's the right number. I do know infections remain a big problem for medical care. They are one reason to think twice about surgery, about procedures, and about hospitalization in general. They are another reason why action is not reliably the safer choice.

IT'S NOT JUST ABOUT INFECTION

The only time I've had anything vaguely resembling surgery was when I was a college student and had my wisdom teeth removed. I felt fine; I was told they "had" to come out to prevent future problems. Maybe I avoided a future problem, but I definitely developed an immediate one. I felt really sick and was kept in the hospital for three days. I was vomiting constantly after surgery—and a lot of what I was vomiting was blood. I don't know exactly what went wrong; I do remember being told that I had had a bad reaction to anesthesia and that I had swallowed too much blood. As I write that, it almost sounds like it was my fault. But that's what I was told.

It is tempting to go off on a tirade about prophylactic wisdom teeth extraction. Sure, millions of wisdom teeth are removed from asymptomatic patients every year in the United States. Of course, there are a lot of strong opinions about the need to do this, although there are very little data supporting this approach. And yes, those institutions that review data and provide guidance—like the UK's National Institute for Health and Care Excellence and the American Public Health Association—recommend that wisdom teeth not be removed prophylactically and should only be removed in patients who are experiencing problems.

But I'm not a dentist. If you're one, you already know that the topic of too much dentistry could fill a whole book. Write it.

I was being teed up for a bigger operation. An oral surgeon thought I should have my malocclusion fixed. My problem was an open bite: only my molars made contact when my jaw was closed. My upper and lower front teeth didn't overlap; instead there was a big gap. I could take a bite out of a sandwich, but the lettuce would always be left behind. I had been subjected to braces and bands with little effect, and now I was being told I needed a real operation.

The oral surgeon would cut my mandible—the lower jawbone—on both sides. He would then reattach it at a more favorable angle so my front teeth would overlap when I took a bite. Made sense. He did mention I would be on a liquid diet for six weeks—as he would need to wire my jaw closed to allow the bone to heal.

I was just a college kid, twenty years old. I was spending my summers working as a paramedic in Boulder County. When you work on an ambulance, there's a lot of attention given to maintaining an open airway—making sure there is nothing to obstruct the flow of air into a patient's lungs. And I had just spent a lot of time vomiting following surgery. So it was natural for me to ask how I would keep my airway clear if for some reason I vomited while recovering from surgery—given that my jaw would be wired shut.

Not to worry, he said. They always made sure wire cutters were available on the bed stand.

I didn't need to consult my parents. The prospect of post-op vomiting, not being able to open my mouth, having to find some wire cutters—not to mention finding the wires to cut—and then opening a jaw that had just been broken (*can you say, pain?*) was sufficient. Inaction was for me. So my teeth still don't close all the way. But it's not like I've had a problem maintaining my weight . . .

Infection is not the only reason to think twice about surgical action. As I get older, one of the harms of surgery I'd be most concerned about is impaired cognition (I don't need more of that). There is a subset of patients who are simply "not the same" after major surgery. They can't think as clearly as they could before. While the problem is best documented following cardiac surgery, it can happen after any major surgery, particularly in the elderly. It doesn't seem to matter what type of anesthesia is given. We don't know why it happens, but we have given it a name: *postoperative cognitive dysfunction.*

And mental health isn't the only concern. All surgery entails trauma—some cutting, piercing, or stretching of body tissues—in other words, some immediate damage to the body. That fact is reflected in our language: patients need to "recover" from surgery. To be sure, the human body can heal; many patients recover without problems. But not all.

A PAIN IN THE BACK

The case for surgical inaction is particularly strong for low back pain. Low back pain is an incredibly common problem. In fact, I have some right now—thanks to an overnight snowfall (which I love) and shoveling the walk (which I'm less fond of). Shoveling is hard on backs—I can't imagine how I'd feel if my work involved shoveling a lot of dirt. Fortunately, my wife does all the gardening.

Most back pain is musculoskeletal—meaning it involves connective tissue: muscles, ligaments, and cartilage. The anatomy of the back is extraordinarily complex: a stack of vertebral bones, wired together with multiple layers of connective tissue of varying lengths and varying angles. All back surgery disturbs this tissue—risking the disturbing side effect of turning acute back pain into chronic back pain. For many back pain patients, surgery has done more harm than good.

In 2011, researchers tracked patients in Ohio who had their back pain evaluated because they had been injured at work. The patients were overwhelmingly male, had an average age of forty, and had little formal education (80 percent had a high school education or less). Not surprisingly, their work typically involved moving heavy objects: furniture, appliances, bulk groceries, car parts, and alcoholic beverages. (I never buy a case of bottled beer anymore—too heavy—the twelve-pack was a great innovation).

The researchers compared 725 patients who received back surgery with 725 patients who did not. Let's be clear: this is not a randomized trial, it's observational research—so it is always reasonable to wonder if the two groups differ in ways other than having or not having surgery. But the researchers made considerable efforts to construct otherwise comparable groups: all the patients had a low back injury on the job—and, importantly, no other injury—and the two groups had the same distribution of diagnoses following evaluation (there were five diagnostic categories) as well as the same age, gender, education, and marital status.

Surgery certainly didn't help people get back to work. Two years following the injury, 26 percent of surgical patients were working as compared to 67 percent of those who did not undergo surgery. And for my epidemiology colleagues who are appropriately skeptical about the comparability of these two groups, forget the comparison and just consider the outcomes for the surgical patients: over one-quarter of whom required a second operation (some a third, fourth, or even a fifth). And get this: two years after surgery, over three-quarters were still taking narcotics for back pain!

I think it's safe to say: back surgery doesn't work that well for back pain.

As I said: low back pain is incredibly common. What I didn't mention was, so are anatomic abnormalities of the back—if we look at them by imaging the spine with a CT scan or MRI. Put the two together and there are a lot of folks to potentially operate on. But there's a hitch: the pain and the abnormalities frequently have nothing to do with each other. Even people without back pain have these abnormalities. In other words, fixing the anatomic abnormalities doesn't reliably fix the pain, because the abnormalities aren't reliably the cause of the pain. Add to that the fact that back surgery can cause pain and you understand why repeat operations account for a substantial portion of all back surgery.

And one surgeon who provides second opinions recently reported that 14 percent of patients scheduled for back surgery in Manhattan didn't even have anatomic abnormalities of the back. . . .

The overuse of back surgery in the United States has been a concern for years. Last time someone checked, we did back surgery at twice the rate of other developed countries—and at five times the rate of the United Kingdom. But even within the United States, my colleagues at the *Dartmouth Atlas* have shown that your chance of having back surgery is highly dependent on where you live. Amazingly, Manhattan is toward the low end of the spectrum. If you live in Boise, your chance is four times higher—maybe it's something about digging up potatoes (or, perhaps, digging post holes for ranch fencing). Check that: Fort Meyers, Florida, has about the same rate of back surgery as Boise—so maybe it's also something about lying on the sand (or, perhaps, carrying heavy binoculars for bird watching on nearby Sanibel Island). But the more likely explanation has nothing to do with the patients and everything to do with the doctors—specifically the number of spine surgeons. Back surgery—to say the least—is all over the map.

But I'd caution you not to raise too many questions about back surgery. Two decades ago one of my colleagues reviewed the research on spinal fusion surgery and concluded there was no evidence of benefit, but there was evidence of substantial complications. That prompted an aggressive attack from the spine surgeons. And the attack wasn't simply directed at him; their lobbying nearly led to the demise of the small federal agency that supports research to figure out what works in medical care. Money matters.

By a quirk of institutional history, the teaching assistants assigned to my undergraduate course have been ortho residents—physicians who are in the midst of their specialty training in orthopedic surgery (which is all about bones, joints, and backs . . .). I feel fortunate: they've been great to work with and the Dartmouth students love them. In addition to having a bunch of other duties, each gives a lecture on orthopedics.

The ortho residents never want to talk to the Dartmouth students about back surgery. They know the facts that patients undergoing surgery typically require subsequent narcotics and frequently require reoperation serve as powerful evidence that current surgical practice causes at least as many problems as it solves. They know there is way too much back surgery going on in the United States and that current practice is all over the map. And they know that some of their orthopedic forebearers have been more focused on financial self-interest than the interests of their patients.

Of course, the ortho residents know these things; they are being trained at Dartmouth. The CEO and president of Dartmouth-Hitchcock Medical Center is an orthopedic spine surgeon who has been questioning back surgery for decades. And Dartmouth Medical School is all about asking hard questions about medical care.

So it is understandable that the ortho residents want to talk to students about what is arguably the biggest success story in orthopedics: joint replacements (a topic for the next chapter). They don't want to talk about back surgery—it is not a fun, or easy, story to tell. One of them was fond of saying, "*Back surgery should only be done on patients who don't have back pain*"—reflecting the observation that the problem best addressed by back surgery is nerve compression, which is typically manifested by pain in the leg or buttock, not pain in the back.

For many of us, back pain is a part of life. While it can knock you off your feet, it almost always gets better with time—particularly when you make the effort to get back on your feet. Minimizing back pain is less about taking surgical action and more about general conditioning, warming up, lifting technique, and knowing when to get mechanical (and human) help. Back surgery is not a panacea; it's an invasive operation.

WHAT ABOUT MINIMALLY INVASIVE SURGERY?

Because everyone acknowledges that surgery produces some up-front trauma, there has been great interest in reducing that damage—using so-called minimally invasive surgery. Conventional surgery requires long skin incisions for two reasons: (1) so surgeons can see what they are doing and (2) so they can introduce their tools—the surgical instruments for grasping, cutting, clamping, sewing, etc. Minimally invasive surgery, therefore, required two technologic leaps. The first was the advent of small-diameter optical devices—laproscopes, arthroscopes—that could be passed through a small incision to allow the surgeon to see well (requiring well-focused light and the ability to produce a magnified image). The second was the advent of small surgical instruments that could be passed through a similarly small incision.

Minimally invasive surgery is a real advance; it reduces the amount of trauma caused by surgery. That means individual patients are subjected to less harm. The problem is that it also reduces the threshold to perform the surgery. That means more people are operated on.

In a classic study of surgery in the state of Maryland during the early 1990s, investigators examined the effect of the introduction of minimally invasive gall bladder surgery. The conventional surgery to remove a gall bladder was a big operation: in some patients the incision could be as long as a foot (some of you might remember the 1960s picture of Lyndon Johnson displaying his scar to the White House press corps). The new minimally invasive surgery required only four small holes. As expected, the investigators found that patients undergoing the minimally invasive surgery were much less likely to die than those undergoing the conventional procedure. But they also found that the number of deaths from gall bladder surgery had not changed in Maryland.

How can that be? It's because the advent of minimally invasive surgery led to so many more gall bladders being taken out.

Ironically, the less invasive surgery becomes, the less carefully we think about it. As the harms are minimized, it tends to distract us from the central question: Does the surgery produce benefit?

In the case of arthroscopic surgery of the knee, too often the answer is no. Arthroscopic surgery is minimally invasive surgery. Before arthroscopic surgery, surgeons opened the entire knee—with an incision four to six inches long. Recovery times were usually measured in months. With arthroscopic surgery, surgeons make a few small holes—one for the arthroscope and one or two for the surgical instruments used in the knee joint. Recovery times are now often measured in weeks. That has lowered the threshold to do the surgery and the number of procedures has skyrocketed.

In 2002, VA investigators performed a radical experiment: veterans with knee arthritis were randomized to either receive arthroscopic surgery or not. And they were very careful to make sure that patients randomized not to receive surgery didn't know that. Here's what happened to that group, after they had been administered a short-acting intravenous tranquilizer:

> To preserve blinding in the event that patients in the placebo group did not have total amnesia, a standard arthroscopic debridement procedure was simulated. After the knee was prepped and draped, three 1-cm incisions were made in the skin. The surgeon asked for all instruments and manipulated the knee as if arthroscopy were being performed. Saline was splashed to simulate the sounds of lavage. No instrument entered the portals for arthroscopy. The patient was kept in the operating room for the amount of time required for a debridement. Patients spent the night after the procedure in the hospital and were cared for by nurses who were unaware of the treatment-group assignment.

In other words, the placebo group received sham surgery—a trip to the OR with all its accouterments, including the skin incisions. But nothing was done to the knee itself.

So what did the study find? No difference between arthroscopic and sham surgery. Patients in both groups got better.

OK, this was just one study—and it was from the VA. But in 2008 it was repeated in Canada, and researchers there got the same result.

OK, it's just two studies—and they were from some VA in Texas and western Ontario for god's sake. But in May 2013, the study was repeated in US academic medical centers at Harvard, Boston University, Washington University (St. Louis), Rush University, the Mayo Clinic, the Cleveland Clinic, and the center of the universe for everything orthopedic—the Hospital for Special Surgery in New York City. Plus, the study was limited to patients with a clear anatomic knee problem—a meniscal tear—and researchers got the same result.

I was going to stop there. But very recently Finnish orthopedists wanted to get their two bits in. Once again, arthroscopic surgery proved to be no better than sham surgery. And the Finns had to get in this dig on the good ole US of A:

> Approximately 700,000 arthroscopic partial meniscectomies are performed annually in the United States alone, with annual direct medical costs estimated at $4 billion.

Good. I'm not the only one who should get flagged for unnecessary roughness.

As always, there is more nuance. Another one of my orthopedic teaching assistants pointed out something I missed in the Finnish study (it is always tough on me when the student becomes the teacher . . .). Before randomization, all patients had a diagnostic arthroscopy: an examination of the joint using an arthroscope. To see the inside of a joint, you need to enlarge the space by putting in a fluid, in this case a saline solution. Fluid that is put into the joint also comes out, essentially washing out the joint. That's called lavage and is often considered a type of surgery. So, one might argue that the Finnish study compared one type of surgery to another. But then again, I didn't fully describe the surgery group in the VA study. It was actually composed of two subgroups: surgery involving cutting/scraping and surgery only involving lavage. And surgery only involving a lavage didn't help people either. . . .

Confused? Welcome to the evidence base for clinical medicine. Studies are often not directly comparable to one another—the patients are not exactly the same, the interventions are not exactly the same, the outcome measures are not the same. A certain amount of judgment is always required.

My judgment is this: arthroscopic surgery of the knee has been grossly overused in the United States. Ditto for back surgery. These surgeries shouldn't be banned; they should be moderated. We are in the midst of a course correction—recognizing that the benefit of arthroscopic surgery is primarily for acute knee injuries, not chronic knee pain, and that the benefit of back surgery is limited to highly selected patients. But as was the case for the germ theory of disease and the value of antiseptic techniques in surgery, these are course corrections that will be measured in decades.

Just because it's minimally invasive doesn't mean action is called for.

INACTION = ALLOWING THE BODY TO HEAL

One of my colleagues who reviewed this chapter was reminded of a comment made by one of his mentors, "Surgery is for other people." Amusing, but a little extreme. So don't misunderstand me: I'm not saying you should never have surgery. I can imagine situations in which I'd gladly sign the consent form. But I'll always consider the option of inaction.

The reason is that the human body has a remarkable ability to heal. And inaction is a strategy that allows that healing to take place. But don't confuse inaction with inactivity. We know bed rest doesn't help back pain; it tends to make it worse. Moderate activity tends to promote healing, particularly for chronic musculoskeletal pain.

The fact that healing without intervention is possible can be lost on a highly medicalized society. Some problems will disappear on their own. Others persist, but we adapt to them—and feel better. And still others wax and wane. Ironically, medical care may obscure our capacity to heal: people who have a problem seek care—and get better. These stories of "success" lead us to conclude that healing was not possible without medical care.

Imagine that a trusted adviser told you that the world was going to end—unless you took an action. The action recommended is easy to do and has no apparent downsides. You do it—and the world doesn't end. Do you conclude the action works? Do you tell your friends to do it?

Unfortunately such faulty logic is common in medical care. Survivor stories following early cancer detection are one variant of these success stories; patient testimonials on the benefit of treatment are another.

The trade-off between action and inaction is probably easiest to understand in surgery. Whatever benefits are associated with a surgical intervention, those actions are also associated with obvious harms—the risk of infection, cognitive dysfunction, and physical injury.

The question of whether or not to take action is every bit as relevant to surgery today as it was in Garfield's day. In trauma surgery, Dr. Trunkey argues that the fundamental question is this: Does the patient need surgical intervention—with its attendant risk of harm? Or can the body heal itself?

Those surgeons who perform major surgeries may understand the case for inaction better than most doctors. To be sure, as with any generalization, there are exceptions. Some surgeons have a very low threshold to operate, their maxim being "a chance to cut is a chance to cure." But many consider the question of whether or not to operate quite carefully.

There are good reasons for surgeons to consider inaction more carefully than others. Their interventions are more invasive. When things go wrong, they tend to go wrong quickly—and catastrophically. The proximity of intervention and harm makes cause and effect obvious; the magnitude of the harm fosters more caution. And surgeons have all had to explain their thinking in front of their colleagues in surgical morbidity and mortality conferences following a surgical death or calamity. That has a way of making one even more cautious.

Of course they make mistakes. And in both directions. Sometimes they operate when they shouldn't; sometimes they don't operate when they should. But they are trained to always consider that balance.

The rest of us doctors may not be so attentive to that balance. Our interventions are less invasive: prescribe a medicine, order a test, make a referral, and admit to the hospital. Things certainly go wrong, but it may take a while and the resulting problems are typically less dramatic. Cause and effect is less obvious; often there is an interceding cascade of events involving a variety of individuals—witness Mr. Nadeau's cascade in the introduction. That makes it more difficult to ascribe a harm to a single individual, making a single decision.

That tends to makes the rest of us a little less cautious.

OUR PROCLIVITY FOR ACTION

The idea of taking action is very compelling. It's important to explore why.

The most obvious force promoting action is money. Many physicians are paid fee-for-service—the more they do, the more they are paid. Financial interests can be strong. In the business of private practice medicine, the relationship between volume and income is described in darkly humorous terms: "you eat what you kill." But even if the physicians are not paid fee-for-service, the hospitals they work for are. The hospitals express their financial interests to their physicians by measuring (and rewarding) physician "productivity," thus providing the same incentive: do more.

Patients who have paid for comprehensive insurance may also have a financial interest in action. They want to get their money's worth.

But it's not all about money. And it's not all about lawyers, who—whether rightly or wrongly—can punish us for both action and inaction.

There are other motivating forces that drive physicians and patients toward action.

Patients feel heard: Doing something concrete—whether ordering a test, prescribing a medicine, performing a procedure, or making a referral—can make patients feel heard and cared for. Sure there are better ways to do that, but it requires good physician-patient communication. In fact, doing something concrete may be a way for physicians to compensate for poor communication skills. But it's a poor substitute for establishing a genuine connection, which means allowing patients' concerns to be heard and bearing witness to their suffering.

Patients feel better: No matter what we do, patients feel better when we do something—particularly when something is labeled as "treatment." It's called the placebo effect. It's the reason so many antibiotics are prescribed for patients with viral infections (no finger pointing here; I've certainly given my share of unnecessary antibiotics). For viral infections, antibiotics are no better than a placebo pill in making patients feel better. But a placebo pill is typically better than nothing.

Credit for cure: We like taking credit for the success story. For most illness and injuries, the natural course of events—without any medical intervention—is that the patient will get better. Against this backdrop, our actions have a way of looking good. The problem is exemplified in what a teaching colleague told me before I started medical school: "Whenever I have a cold, I get antibiotics from the school doctor and I get better."

Credit for trying: Patients don't always get better; bad things do happen. Doctors and patients alike may experience less regret about these bad things following an effort to do something than they do after failing to do something. I think that's why obituaries so often incorporate the phrase "fought a courageous battle." Doctors, families, and patients all like to be able to say, "At least we tried."

PRESCRIPTION: CONSIDER THE OPTION OF DOING NOTHING

Where there is a problem, there is pressure to do something: Prescribe a medicine. Order a test. Refer to a specialist. Admit to the hospital. Perform an operation. The pressure to do something reflects a belief that action is preferable to inaction. But the reality is that the human body can heal and that all of our actions have unintended consequences. Thus, inaction can often be the preferred course.

Oddly enough, the value of inaction is increasingly recognized in personal finance. Jack Bogle, the founder of the Vanguard investment management group, offered individuals a passive investment strategy: regular savings—with reinvestment of dividends—in a low-cost mutual fund designed to track the stock market as a whole. He recognized that active investors (and mutual fund managers) typically had worse returns than the market average because they could not reliably pick winners and had a tendency to trade in reaction to market swings: selling when the market was low (because it had been falling), buying when the market was high (because it had been rising). While Wall Street benefited from the fees associated with frequent trading, fees only further diminished the returns for the investor. Mr. Bogle's advice was simple:

"Don't just do something. Sit there."

You don't want a knee-jerk recommendation from your financial adviser that you always need to move money around. Any more than you want a knee-jerk recommendation from your insurance agent that you always need to increase coverage. Or from your lawyer that you always need to change the will. Or from your vet that your dog always need shots. Or from your dentist that you always need X-rays. True professionals provide considered advice. And sometimes doing nothing is exactly the right thing to do.

The same is true of medicine. The good doctor is not the one who routinely recommends action. It's too easy for the physician—and it's too easy for you to get somewhere you don't want to be. Recognize that the doctor who advises no action may be the one who really cares for you.

Inaction provides your body the opportunity to heal. It provides time. The passage of time can have both diagnostic and therapeutic value. Most doctors recognize this, but for the reasons outlined above, they may feel compelled to act. To counterbalance this tendency, your strategy should be to pose a simple question: *What happens if I do nothing?*

NEWER IS ALWAYS BETTER

*Disturbing truth: New interventions are
typically not well tested and often wind up
being judged ineffective (even harmful)*

> "For the 86th time in the last 75 years, Procter
> & Gamble has announced New, Improved Tide."

OR SO READ THE OPENING line of an article on thespoof.com. Sure it's an overstatement. And don't think I'm going to beat up on Tide—it was the laundry detergent my mom used to get the grass stains off of my pants when I was a kid.

I don't know the origin of the slogan "new and improved," but Procter & Gamble would be a pretty good bet. P&G has a storied history: founded by a candle maker (Procter) and a soap maker (Gamble), it introduced a series of products that are now household names: Ivory "the soap that floats," Crisco, Crest, Pampers, and, of course, Tide. The company pioneered the use of radio advertising—and is the source of the term "soap opera." And it was advertising on television well before most Americans had one. For business students learning about advertising and branding, P&G is a classic case.

We've all learned to be a little skeptical about the value of newness in household goods. How much better can Tide be made anyway? We may need, however, to apply lessons learned from claims about household products to claims about medical care. In medical care, too often the word *new* is associated with the word *improved*—when it would be better associated with the word *untested*.

A NEW DRUG

In the early 1950s, Grünenthal—a German pharmaceutical company—developed and patented a drug they branded under the trade name Contergan. It was a sedative/hypnotic agent—a drug used to relieve anxiety and induce sleep. The company's website provides a translation of a wistful advertisement for the new drug:

> A moment replete with natural harmony makes us wish the seconds would expand. But it usually remains no more than a moment and a fleeting desire, because the restlessness once useful to the mind dominates us and causes us to roam.

Good hook—even six decades later. If I have a brush with natural harmony, I'd like to stay there for more than a moment. How do I do it?

> Contergan gives peace and sleep. This harmless medicine does not burden the liver metabolism, affects neither blood pressure nor circulation, and is well tolerated even by sensitive patients. Sleep and peace: Contergan, Contergan forte.

Sleep and peace sounds good now—and apparently sounded good then. Contergan was made available over the counter in Germany and became a very successful drug, with sales of more than twelve million marks annually by 1960 (about $30 million in current US dollars).

The drug was a new competitor for the then-standard class of sedative/hypnotic drugs, the barbiturates. Barbiturates—like phenobarbital and secobarbital—pose real problems: they are hard on the liver, they are addictive, and they are easy to overdose. Furthermore, overdose can easily lead to death, either accidentally or purposefully. Contergan apparently offered a new level of safety: it was well tolerated, not habit-forming, and had little potential for misuse as a suicidal agent.

In 1958, the new drug crossed the English Channel and was licensed in the United Kingdom by the Distillers Company. Here it was branded under the trade name Distaval. Instead of promoting sleep and peace, Distillers emphasized the safety of the drug. A dramatic ad featured an unattended toddler opening a bottle of pills with the headline "*This child's life may depend on the safety of Distaval.*" The text went on:

> Consider the possible outcome in a case such as this—had the bottle contained a conventional barbiturate. Year by year, the barbiturates claim a mounting toll of childhood victims. Yet it is simple enough to prescribe a sedative and hypnotic which is both highly effective . . . and outstandingly safe. . . . Distaval has been prescribed for over three years in this country, where the accidental poisonings rate is notoriously high; but there is no case on record in which even gross overdosage with Distaval has had harmful results. Put your mind at rest. Depend on the safety of Distaval.

OK, avoiding death from accidental overdose sounds good too. The new drug was considered so safe it could be claimed to be a wonder drug. And its indications were extended beyond anxiety and sleeplessness to include cough, colds, headaches, and even the morning sickness that often accompanies pregnancy.

> Distaval can be given with complete safety to pregnant women and nursing mothers without adverse effect on mother or child . . .

The drug was ultimately sold in a total of forty-six countries by various pharmaceutical companies under a variety of trade names. Branding may be good for P&G and pharmaceutical companies, but it is sure hard on doctors: multiple trade names make pharmacology so much harder to learn. How would I know that Contergan™ (in Germany) and Distaval™ (in England) are the same drug? A drug has just one generic name. Furthermore, a generic name also often identifies a drug's class: I know phenobarbital, secobarbital, and anything-else-barbital must all be in the barbiturate class. I've always disliked trade names because they add unnecessary confusion. Generic names provide more useful information.

So let's cut to the chase. What is the generic name of this new, safe, and natural harmony-inducing drug?

Thalidomide. Doesn't sound so good anymore. Thalidomide might have been easy on the liver, but it was tough on the fetus. If you were exposed to any visual media during the early 1960s, you probably saw the images of legless and armless toddlers. With a missing arm, for example, the child was typically left with its hands or digits sprouting from the top of the shoulder. It's hard to know what adjective to attach to these images: appalling, tragic, or inexcusable.

When taken early in pregnancy—when arms, legs, and organs are forming—thalidomide causes birth defects. The most common—and the most obvious—were limb defects, but the drug also caused problems to the eyes, the ears, the heart, the liver, the genitals, and the gastro-intestinal tract. Some ten thousand to twenty thousand children were affected worldwide, many of whom died. In Germany alone Grünenthal estimates five thousand children were born with deformities; in the United Kingdom, the corresponding number was about two thousand.

In the United States it was under twenty.

I know it's not fashionable to say anything good about the federal government, but the thalidomide story is arguably one of the finest hours for the US Food and Drug Administration. Not only did the FDA save the William S. Merrell Company from paying millions in damages (as were paid by Grünenthal and Distillers), it helped the country avoid what *Time* labeled the "Thalidomide Disaster."

The hero of the story was a forty-six-year-old woman who had been at the FDA for all of one month when Merrell's new drug approval application for thalidomide hit her desk. She was both a pharmacologist and a physician. And, oddly enough, this American hero was a Canadian.

Frances Oldham Kelsey was disturbed by the observation that large amounts of the drug could be given to animals without producing drowsiness (remember the drug is a sedative/hypnotic). She did not approve the new drug; she wanted more testing. A few months later she learned about the other common side effect of thalidomide, polyneuropathy, or nerve damage to the hands and feet. A few months after that, reports of birth defects appeared from both Germany and Australia. And the rest is history.

As I said, time is useful. It can help distinguish whether "new" really is "improved."

NEW DRUGS AND THE FDA

Paracelsus was a Swiss-German Renaissance physician and alchemist— among other things, as always seems to be the case with Renaissance figures. He authored the classic line of toxicology: "All things are poison, and nothing is without poison; only the dose permits something not to be poisonous."

The statement is certainly true for pharmaceutical agents. Dose matters. But, as the thalidomide story makes clear, dose is not the whole story. Whether a drug is "poisonous" is also a function of who the patient is—and whether she is pregnant. I have a patient on thalidomide. It's not because he suffers from anxiety, insomnia, cough, cold, headaches, or morning sickness—it's because he has multiple myeloma (a relatively rare blood-borne cancer). The FDA approved thalidomide for treating multiple myeloma in 2006, after first approving the drug for a form of leprosy in 1998 (*erythema nodosum leprosum*). So, while it is tempting to think of thalidomide as a dangerous drug, the truth is more nuanced.

The FDA reviews new drugs before they go to market and strives to keep dangerous ones off the market. But it wasn't always this way. In 1937, no requirement for FDA approval existed, and a new preparation of a sulfa antibiotic (elixir sulfanilamide) entered the market. It contained diethylene glycol—a solvent for dyes, oils, and other organic compounds—and over one hundred people died from it. The FDA responded quickly to limit the damage, finding and collecting the remaining supplies of the drug. This was the event that paved the way for the FDA to examine new drugs *before* they were marketed.

It's not an easy job; it's a balancing act. And they can't please everybody. After the thalidomide disaster, the FDA gained new powers and there were complaints they were making too many demands on pharmaceutical manufacturers. Then the United States entered an era of deregulation, and there were complaints that the FDA wasn't doing its job. And the pendulum may be swinging again. It's a delicate balance: how do you keep dangerous new drugs off the market without raising prohibitive hurdles that would also keep good new drugs off the market?

Let's be clear: sometimes new drugs really are improved. In the early 1980s, rare infections (Pnuemocystis carinii pneumonia and cytomegalovirus) and a rare cancer (Kaposi's sarcoma) were found to occur in young gay men. Despite treatment, all died within two years of diagnosis. Their diagnosis was labeled "acquired immune deficiency syndrome"—better known as AIDS—and by 1994 more than 150,000 Americans had died from the disease. Then a new class of pharmacologic agents called protease inhibitors was approved. These agents interfered with the ability of the HIV virus to replicate itself and had a dramatic effect: among young men, the death rate from AIDS plummeted by 75 percent. These drugs turned a deadly infection into a chronic infection—and even led to some cures.

That's a damn good new drug.

But FDA approval is not a guarantee of safety. The FDA has approved drugs that are subsequently withdrawn from the market because of safety concerns. In 1999, they approved a new nonsteroidal anti-inflammatory agent—an aspirin-like drug for arthritis. But no one really thought it was any better at treating pain than over-the-counter drugs like Motrin, Advil, or Midol (all trade names for the drug ibuprofen) or Naprosyn, Anaprox, or Aleve (all trade names for the drug naproxen). *Don't you just hate trade names?*

The only plausible advantage to this new drug was a lower risk of stomach bleeding. But the effect is so small that it probably only applies to those individuals at a very high risk of bleeding. Oh ... and I guess it had one other advantage from the manufacturers' perspective: it could be sold for ten to fifty times the cost of its over-the-counter generic competitors. Thanks to effective direct-to-consumer marketing, over twenty million Americans took the new drug.

Until it was pulled off the market in 2004 because it caused heart attacks and strokes.

That's the Vioxx story—and it is not unique. The website *Worst Pills, Best Pills* lists twenty drugs approved by the FDA in 1993 or later that were subsequently withdrawn:

> Of the 20 drugs, two were antibiotics: grepafloxacin (RAXAR) and gatifloxacin (TEQUIN); three were nonsteroidal anti-inflammatory drugs: bromfenac (DURACT), rofecoxib (VIOXX) and valdecoxib (BEXTRA); two drugs were for weight loss: sibutramine and dexfenfluramine (REDUX); and one was for type-2 diabetes: troglitazone (REZULIN). Another diabetes drug, rosiglitazone (AVANDIA) recently has had some restrictions on its use but unlike in Europe, where it was completely banned, it is still being used in the U.S.

Sorry, that's a lot of names (TRADENAMES).

Why are so many drugs withdrawn from the market *after* being approved by the FDA? It's not necessarily because the FDA is asleep at the wheel (although it can be). It's because it takes time to get the big picture—to learn the full range of a drug's effects. Sidney Wolfe, the founder of the website *Worst Pills, Best Pills*, summarized the problem this way:

> New drugs are tested in a relatively small number of people before being released, and serious adverse effects or life-threatening drug interactions may not be detected until the new drug has been taken by hundreds of thousands of people.

Actually there are two explanations for why it takes time to learn the full range of a drug's effect. The first is about the numbers: new drug approval is based on testing relatively few, while safety issues may only become evident after the drug has been given to many. The second is about the patients. New drug approval is usually based on testing performed in a select group of patients: they are relatively healthy and only have the disease for which the drug is being tested. And they are only taking one medication. After approval, however, the new drug is given to a broad array of patients: older, sicker, with a variety of other diseases—and patients who take multiple medications. These patients are deliberately not included in pre-approval drug testing.

For these reasons, Dr. Wolfe advocates a "7-year rule": unless the drug is one of those rare "breakthroughs"—like protease inhibitors were for AIDS—you want to wait seven years from the date of release before taking a new drug.

I don't know if seven is the right number; I do know that time adds to our knowledge. Remember Huey Lewis and the News? In 1984, they released the single "I Want a New Drug." But I don't want a new drug; I want an old drug. Not one that is outdated, mind you, but one that has been road-tested—one that's been around for a while.

A NEW PROCEDURE—A QUANTUM LEAP

Let me now share a quantum leap forward in medical care—followed by a leap of faith that ultimately put thousands of women through hell.

First, some context for the quantum leap. The clinical context is the disease leukemia—a blood-borne cancer, like multiple myeloma. Fifty years ago, the diagnosis of leukemia was a death sentence. The treatment context is radiation and chemotherapy. For most cancers, the first-line strategy is to cut the cancer out with surgery. But in leukemia, and the other blood-borne cancers, there is nothing to cut out—the cancer is disseminated throughout the body. That's where radiation and chemotherapy come in. Both tend to kill rapidly dividing cells, like cancer cells. The problem is that they also kill cells that normally divide rapidly—like the cells that make blood in the bone marrow. It's a problem that limits their dose: how much radiation and chemotherapy doctors can safely give cancer patients.

A crazy idea surfaced in the late 1950s. What about giving a leukemia patient very high doses of radiation and chemotherapy—doses that would kill the cancer, kill the marrow, and kill the patient—but then "rescue" the patient by transplanting bone marrow from a healthy donor?

Who had this crazy idea? It was a Texan—one of those folks who think big. He grew up during the Depression. His father was a solo general practitioner who made house calls in a horse and buggy. His family was poor—GPs didn't make much money before the advent of health insurance—but so were most of his father's patients. The son hunted and fished for food. He was not an outstanding student, even among his 1936 high school graduating class of fifteen. He went to the University of Texas to study chemistry and chemical engineering and began to catch fire. He was admitted to Harvard Medical School and did research at Harvard hospitals for nearly a decade.

But the idea was too crazy for Harvard. He needed to break out of the box—out of the confines of an academic medical center—and found an employer eager to have him push the idea forward. It was in the middle of nowhere: specifically, in Cooperstown, New York. By 1957 he had tried out the crazy idea on six patients with advanced leukemia at the Mary Imogene Bassett Hospital. It was a spectacular failure: all had died within one hundred days.

Yet in 1990 Edward Donnall Thomas was in Stockholm to receive the Nobel Prize.

Of course, a lot had to happen in between. Dr. Thomas moved from Cooperstown to the University of Washington during the 1960s to refine the new procedure. It wasn't easy. He had to persevere through multiple early failures—and he had to ignore the suggestions of colleagues that he give up on the idea.

I was fortunate enough to work with Dr. Thomas briefly in the late 1980s and was struck to see such a renowned physician wearing cowboy boots in an academic hospital. But it worked—this was a guy who had to challenge a lot of medical conventions.

The challenge wasn't the surgical technique of marrow transplantation—that part is easy: bone marrow is a liquid that can be infused into a vein. So giving someone bone marrow cells is like giving someone blood—or an IV fluid. The challenge is what happens next: an immunological nightmare. Hospital stays were measured in weeks. Too little immune function and patients develop (and die from) unusual infections; too much immune function and patients develop diseases in which the immune system starts attacking the body itself. To avoid infection, patients have to be isolated in special laminar airflow rooms; to avoid immune self-attack, patients have to be immunosuppressed. It was a delicate balance, with very high stakes.

Dr. Thomas was responsible for a quantum leap in medicine—the development of bone marrow transplantation. Bone marrow transplantation is now commonplace in the treatment of leukemia and is an important part of the explanation for why it is no longer necessarily a death sentence.

A NEW PROCEDURE—A LEAP OF FAITH

Given the success of marrow transplantation in treating cancers of the blood (representing only about 10 percent of all cancers), it is not surprising that someone would want to try the procedure on one of the so-called "solid tumors" (the remaining 90 percent of cancers). The prime candidate was breast cancer.

By the late 1980s, there were strong proponents for using marrow transplantation for advanced breast cancer. And they weren't shy about sharing their beliefs about the new procedure with the press, as exemplified by a story in the *Los Angeles Times*:

> A combination of bone marrow transplants and very high doses of anticancer drugs may be able to double the survival rate of patients with advanced breast cancer, a Boston researcher reported last week.

But there were no data to support such statements. What data existed came from case reports—reports showing that some women had cancer shrinkage following the procedure. Having your cancer become smaller sounds like a good thing, but it often has no bearing on how good you feel—or how long you live. To know if a procedure really helps patients, we need to compare those who get the procedure with those who don't—in a randomized trial.

Bone marrow transplantation for breast cancer became a big news story. There may not have been much data, but there were many interesting angles: a deadly disease that could affect young mothers with children, an innovative and technologically advanced procedure, an enormous price tag of about $100,000, and even a villain—greedy insurance companies.

It all came together in 1990 when the *Washington Post* ran the headline "Maryland Mother's Chance of Life Hinges on Trial; Patient Sues Insurers For Cancer Treatment Cost." Pamela Pirozzi—a thirty-five-year-old mother of three—had been advised that her best chance of surviving more than a year was a transplant, but her insurance company had refused coverage, stating the procedure was still "experimental." Armed with a list of insurance companies in other states that, when challenged, had agreed to pay for the procedure, the Pirozzis sued. A federal judge ruled in Pamela Pirozzi's favor, writing:

> To require that the plaintiff or other plan members wait until somebody chooses to present statistical proof . . . that would satisfy all the experts means that plan members would be doomed to receive medical procedures that are not state of the art.

It was a bad decision: it equated new—"state of the art"—with improved. But the same mistake was being made across the country: women who were dying of breast cancer were being told bone marrow transplantation was their best chance, and insurers who failed to pay for the procedure were being compelled to by federal courts—or the court of public opinion.

The stories were tragic—both for the women and the insurers. Nelene Fox—a thirty-nine-year-old California mother of three—was diagnosed with breast cancer in 1991 and soon found to have metastatic disease. Her insurer, Health Net, refused her request for a transplant, stating it did not cover "investigational" procedures. With the aid of 1,700 donors, Ms. Fox's family raised $210,000. She underwent the treatment in 1992 and died a few months later. Her husband and brother (an attorney) sued Health Net for their refusal to pay, and the jury ruled in favor of the family. The 1993 award, $89.1 million, was the largest ever levied against an insurance company for refusing to provide health coverage benefits.

Not surprisingly, that led a lot of insurance companies simply to give in to demands to pay for the procedure.

For the remaining holdouts, a new opponent appeared: the federal government. Luckily I just wrote something nice about it, because it didn't look so good here. In September 1994, the Office of Personnel Management ordered all health plans serving federal employees to grant coverage of bone marrow transplantation for breast cancer within twenty-four hours or risk being dropped from the program. The decision affected 350 health plans serving nine million people.

It was another bad decision: why did they do that? Political pressure was certainly part of the story—a year earlier, fifty-four members of Congress wrote to demand that the Office of Personnel Management cover the procedure. They cited statistics from a report at Duke University claiming transplantation and high dose chemotherapy were "eight times more effective than conventional dose therapy."

New and *eight* times better. Never heard that claim before. Closest I've got is a Tresemme shampoo bottle—made by Unilever, one of P&G's major competitors—that says it is *five* times smoother and silkier . . .

A lot of that political pressure was coming from academic medical centers that were beginning to make real money off the procedure. Breast cancer is a much bigger market than leukemia and quickly became the most common reason for performing the procedure. Academic medical centers had set up special units just for breast cancer patients. Of course, they were lobbying Congress and presenting extremely favorable data.

Yet another branch of the federal government wasn't so sure—the National Cancer Institute. Their position was made clear in congressional testimony: "Formal scientific evaluation ought to precede the routine use of such a toxic and expensive therapy."

That sounds like prudent advice. It certainly was an expensive therapy: $100,000 was a lot of money in 1990, as it is today (with inflation the current price tag would be about $200,000). And it certainly was a toxic therapy. In fact, the whole point of the bone marrow transplant was so the patient could tolerate what would otherwise be a deadly dose of chemotherapy. The transplant typically kept the patients alive, but it couldn't avoid other toxic effects: women undergoing high dose chemotherapy with transplantation were about ten times more likely than women undergoing conventional chemotherapy to become anemic (69 percent versus 6 percent), to become infected (31 percent versus 3 percent), and to develop serious diarrhea (25 percent versus 1 percent).

Certainly it was important to ask the most basic question: Does it work?

Ironically, all the publicity—and all the politics—made the question harder to address. The presumption of benefit became widespread: being able to give more chemotherapy *must* lead to better outcomes. Investigators struggled to find women willing to participate in randomized trials. Having insurers capitulate and cover the procedure further buttressed presumptions about benefit (if it's covered, it must be effective). And I believe the high price tag only added to the apparent case (anything that is so expensive must be good).

But investigators persisted, and by the turn of the century a very different message prevailed, as summarized in a *New England Journal of Medicine* editorial:

> To a reasonable degree of probability [high-dose chemotherapy and bone marrow transplantation for advanced breast cancer] has been

proved to be ineffective and should be abandoned in favor of well justified alternative experimental approaches.

What happened? Randomized trials had been completed. They showed marrow transplantation had allowed us to make women sicker (by allowing more chemotherapy to be given), but it didn't help women live longer. In 2011 an overview of trials was published in the *Journal of Clinical Oncology* summarizing the evidence:

> Overall survival of patients with metastatic breast cancer in the six randomized trials was not significantly improved by high-dose chemotherapy; any benefit from high doses was small. No identifiable subset of patients seems to benefit from high-dose chemotherapy.

That's a stark conclusion: no one was helped. And the harms of high-dose chemotherapy and marrow transplantation were obvious: women were subjected to more intensive therapies with more intensive toxicities. Extra weeks in the hospital; extra weeks feeling sick—in a group of women who didn't have a lot of extra weeks to waste.

There are actually reasons to be even more cautious about new procedures than new drugs. Prescribing a drug is not technically challenging: it's easy to write a prescription (although spelling the drug's name can be tough). But procedures can be technically challenging, and it can take time for physicians to master them.

In the case of marrow transplantation, what was challenging was not the transplant itself—recall, it is not that different from simply giving blood. What was challenging was learning how to manage all the subsequent complications: infection, bleeding, immune self-attack, etc. During the explosive growth of transplantation for breast cancer, many hospitals opened transplant centers—despite having no prior experience with the procedure. Even the transplant community, those physicians who performed transplants and believed the therapy worked, was worried at the time about the quality of care provided by these new centers. Had the trials been done at these centers, and not the experienced ones, I suspect transplants would have been found to increase mortality.

In the case of other surgical procedures, the challenge is often in the procedure itself or in learning how to use new equipment. Mastering a new technique or a new piece of robotic equipment takes time. Simply put: there is a learning curve for new procedures.

I don't want a new procedure. I want one that is known to work and one my doctor knows how to do.

MEDICAL DEVICES

When I started medical school I had a simple categorization of the therapeutic actions available to doctors—we could either prescribe a drug or perform a procedure. (Here, I'm purposely excluding all the actions related to caring, sharing, reassuring, witnessing, etc.)

But there is a third category that is increasingly relevant: therapeutic actions involving a medical device. In medical care the term "device" encompasses a broad array of equipment, from simple stuff like tongue depressors and bandages to complex machines like respirators and defibrillators. But the new devices that are most relevant to this discussion are those that are implanted inside the human body.

The only implantable device I can remember being discussed in medical school was an intrauterine device, or IUD. At one point IUDs were the preferred form of reversible contraception; now IUDs are undergoing a resurgence. In-between was the Dalkon Shield, an ill-fated IUD that was debatably related to pelvic inflammatory disease and infertility. What is not debatable is the fact that the Dalkon Shield was withdrawn from the market following multiple lawsuits, an episode that discouraged the use of IUDs for decades.

Today, implantable devices are increasingly common—we regularly put artificial lenses in eyes, tubes in ears, and all sorts of stuff in the heart: valves, stents, pacemakers, and defibrillators. But the specialty most associated with implantable hardware is orthopedics, where screws, rods, pins, and plates are routinely placed into bones, and even entire joints are replaced.

A DOCTOR GETS A NEW DEVICE

The general medical officers I worked with in rural Alaska were all young—late twenties, early thirties. That fact juxtaposed with the English verb we commonly use to describe the provision of medical care—"practicing"—created more than a little apprehension in some of the native population we served. After practicing in the bush for a number of years, most of us returned to the Lower 48 for additional training.

After five years in the Indian Health Service, Steve went south to train in orthopedics. He returned to Alaska to do what orthopedists do best: hip and knee replacements. I was reminded by one of the orthopedists who reviewed this chapter that this might not be the most *important* thing they do—that the old standby of fixing broken bones arguably tops that list. Nevertheless, joint replacements represent a major success story in medicine, not because they help people live longer, but because they help people live better, move better, and have less pain.

After about twenty years of orthopedic practice, Steve developed a dull pain on his left side. His pain was hard to localize, but it was somewhere between the groin and buttock. Walking made it worse; running and skiing made it much worse. He stopped running and skiing. Even standing at the operating table began to hurt. Resting helped but didn't take the pain away. Steve began to have pain while doing nothing, like just lying in bed at night. He wasn't sleeping well.

That's a problem for all of us but particularly for surgeons, whom we'd all like to see wide awake. Steve knew he needed the operation he had performed on hundreds of patients. He needed a hip replacement.

A hip replacement involves the implantation of a medical device—an artificial hip implant. A hip implant is actually two pieces of hardware: a ball that is implanted into the top of the femur (the upper leg bone), and a socket that is implanted into the pelvis. The ball fits in the socket—allowing for a broad range of motion. You are born with a ball and socket joint in the hip; the device simply follows the design of your original equipment.

For the mechanically inclined, a hip implant looks a lot like the ball joint connection to the tie rod in your car—the apparatus that allows you to steer (although the hip implant is a whole lot more expensive). One year, when discussing hip replacements in my undergraduate class, we passed around multiple hip implants so that the students could inspect them. I had just had the ball joints replaced on my 1999 Volvo, so I threw one of them into the mix. No one noticed—despite the fact I left a little grease on it—providing evidence that Dartmouth undergrads aren't particularly mechanically inclined.

Not only do hip implants and automotive ball joints share a similar appearance, they share a common problem—both can wear out and fail. That's right, a hip replacement may need to be replaced.

As an orthopedic surgeon, Steve understood this problem better than most. He knew replacing a previously replaced hip was a tough operation. Furthermore, Steve was still young—at least from my vantage point—he was just about to turn fifty. Most of the patients he was performing hip replacements on were in their sixties and seventies. And Steve was active; he was an avid hiker and an endurance biker. He wanted his new hip to last a long time and hold up to some serious wear and tear.

Steve had a lot of hip implants to choose from. I wouldn't be surprised if there are more choices in hip implants than there are in laundry detergents. There is a simple reason for this: the market is huge. There are over 400,000 hip replacements performed each year in the United States alone. According to the "Paying Till It Hurts" series in the *New York Times*, an implant costs about $350 to make but sells to hospitals and clinics for $4,500 to $7,500.

A ten- to twentyfold markup? That's a good business to be in. Given that it's such a good business to be in, you might expect a lot of businesses to be in the business. But there are not: there are only five major players. That's a setup for a cartel—a few firms agreeing on pricing—a moniker recently acquired by P&G and Unilever for price-fixing laundry detergents in Europe.

At least the soap manufacturers don't pay doctors to use their products. The five implant companies accepted federal monitoring in 2007 to avoid criminal prosecution for illegal kickbacks to surgeons. That monitoring revealed in 2008 that the five companies paid over $200 million to about five hundred orthopedic surgeons. Was that to support their important research? Or was it payment for using and promoting a particular implant? We don't know. While there is undoubtedly some important research being done, we do know that over half the surgeons had no academic affiliation—and that even having an academic affiliation is no guarantee that industry support is going toward important research.

It gets worse. The hospitals pay $4,500 to $7,500 for an implant—then add on their own markup. On the itemized bill, the implants can go as high as $37,000. To be fair, the hospitals have other costs: in particular, they are trying to recoup foregone revenues from those patients who underpay. But they are also trying to keep all their orthopedic surgeons happy. Different surgeons like to use different implants. And different implants require different—noncompatible—surgical instruments. That's extra inventory, extra equipment, extra cost, and extra complexity—which is why hospitals engage "joint consultants" and "joint brokers."

There's a lot of money on this table. Not to mention a lot of folks who ought to be wearing cowboy boots—because this is the Wild West of medicine. Constantly changing, apparently differentiated implants (slightly different designs, sizes, and materials), each often requiring a unique "toolkit," that can be bundled—and unbundled. . . . What a great way to obscure prices. That's why Steve had a full range of models to choose from.

Despite this bewildering array of hardware, most hip implants have the same basic design: the ball is metal and the socket is a metal cap lined with a hard plastic. When placed in the human body, the metal ball makes contact with the hard plastic, allowing smooth, relatively frictionless motion. But the plastic begins to wear away with years of use. That's when the hip replacement needs replacing.

In 2005, DePuy introduced its new hip implant: the ASR XL. Pretty cool sounding name, huh? What was new is that they had eliminated the plastic liner. That allowed the ball to be bigger (and, theoretically, less likely to dislocate) and avoided the problem of having the plastic wear away (theoretically, allowing the implant to last longer). Now the metal ball was making contact with the metal cap—leading to the more common term for the new implant: the metal-on-metal hip.

Metal-on-metal was billed as a long-lasting implant designed for active, young patients. It sounded like the perfect implant for Steve. He got one.

A year later Steve didn't feel so well. He had become irritable. He noticed that he couldn't exercise as vigorously as he had in the past. And most disturbing of all, his hip started hurting again. That's not supposed to happen.

Another year passed. Now Steve was frankly depressed. He wondered if that was simply due to the return of his hip pain, but other things were going wrong as well. He could barely exercise because he felt so out of breath. He developed a tremor. His ears were ringing and his hearing seemed to be failing. His vision also seemed to be failing—words would go missing while he was reading, small lights would flash while he was driving at night. Was he going crazy?

No. He was being poisoned.

With each step he took, the metal ball rotated against the metal cap. That rubbing produced metallic debris. These small particles of cobalt and chromium—the alloy used to make the metal-on-metal hip—irritated the surrounding tissue. That's what made the new hip hurt. Cobalt and chromium ions then entered the bloodstream. That's what caused all the other symptoms.

This was not easy to figure out. The prominence of the psychiatric symptoms led Steve's doctors to assume a psychiatric cause. He was irritable, he was excitable, he was depressed, he was manic. Variable moods—he must be bipolar. Steve developed a new sympathy for patients who are given the message: "It's all in your head." (At the same time, acknowledging it's a possibility worth considering in all of us.)

But Steve was in a better position than most to investigate the problem. He was a doctor—he could order tests on himself. Moreover, he was a surgeon. He knew the device and its mechanics; he could imagine what might be going on.

So he ordered a test I didn't even know existed: a serum cobalt level. It was 122 micrograms per liter. Doesn't sound like much, but it's over one hundred times the upper limit of normal.

Of course that doesn't prove that it wasn't all in his head. Maybe he just happens to have high cobalt levels *and* bipolar disorder. But Steve also had physical abnormalities. An audiology examination showed high-frequency hearing loss. An ophthalmology examination showed optic nerve atrophy. And an echocardiogram showed mild heart failure.

About three years after his hip replacement, Steve asked his partner to remove the metal-on-metal implant and replace it with a conventional one. It was a difficult operation: the soft tissues surrounding the hip were swollen and inflamed in reaction to the metal debris. But after it was done, Steve's cobalt levels returned to normal. More importantly, his symptoms resolved.

That's as good as evidence for cause and effect can get in a single patient.

And Steve is not the only case of cobalt poisoning following hip replacement—nor the most severe one. A couple of weeks ago the *Lancet* reported on a fifty-five-year-old man who developed severe heart failure after the head of his metal hip wore down and formed tiny debris. Why did he develop heart failure? Because his cobalt levels were a thousand times normal. The same week, the *New England Journal of Medicine* reported on a fifty-nine-year-old woman who developed such severe heart failure that she required a heart transplant before she was recognized to be suffering from cobalt poisoning from her metal-on-metal hip implants. And before her implants were removed, her transplanted heart showed signs of failing.

That's two hips, damaging two hearts, in the same patient.

You get the picture: high levels of cobalt are hard on the heart. Interestingly, that's not new news. During the 1960s, in both Quebec and Omaha, there were mini-epidemics of rapidly progressive heart failure in young, otherwise healthy individuals. Almost one hundred cases were reported, and nearly half died. But the cobalt didn't come from a medical device; it came from a foam-stabilizing agent used in beer.

No one stabilizes beer foam with cobalt anymore. Lucky for me—or else I'd have to move back home to Colorado to gain ready access to an alternative recreational substance.

Just how common the systemic effects of cobalt poisoning are following metal-on-metal implants is the subject of some debate. It certainly doesn't affect all patients, yet orthopedists are certainly clear on one point: if your metal-on-metal patient develops an unexpected medical problem, checking a cobalt level is a pretty darn good place to start.

There is no debate about the local effects of metal-on-metal hips: the tissue surrounding the implant can be damaged by the reaction to the metal debris. Large collections of fluid may form—as big as a grapefruit. This local reaction even has a name: pseudotumor. The treatment is to remove the pseudotumor and the hardware that caused it.

Metal-on-metal hips were supposed to last longer than conventional implants. But according to the National Joint Registry for England, Wales, and Northern Ireland, they are actually five times more likely than conventional implants to require replacement.

What are the corresponding data for the United States? No one knows. That's because we have so many companies providing insurance—and because a patient's insurance company may change—that it is practically impossible for us to get the big picture for any device (or any procedure—or any drug).

Thanks to the other side of the pond, we know that 20 percent of metal-on-metal hips will fail within nine years of being implanted. To be sure, that means 80 percent do not fail within nine years—it's important to flip the frame, particularly if you have a metal-on-metal hip. Most people do well; most do not develop a pseudotumor.

But make no mistake about it: 20 percent within nine years is a high failure rate. For context, consider the Mayo Clinic experience from 1970 with one of the original hip implants—the Charnley hip. Nowhere near as cool-sounding as the ASR XL—and nowhere near as expensive. It was one of the first implants: nothing fancy, it was made out of stainless steel. Furthermore, the surgeons were just learning how to do the procedure at the time. But it took more than twenty-five years before 20 percent had failed.

How crazy is that? You've got one of the biggest success stories in medicine going on. Why would you change the equipment? Are they trying to make something very good, even better? Or are they trying to sell more product?

That's why Steve says, when it comes to hips, "older is better."

PRESCRIPTION—STICK WITH TRIED-AND-TRUE

No matter how many times Tide has been reintroduced as new and improved, it has remained a really great product. (Full disclosure: This portion of the book has *not* been brought to you by the Procter & Gamble Company, Cincinnati, Ohio.)

But, in general, I remain a little hesitant about the value of newness. I'm not a "first adopter" of new software—there are too many bugs to deal with. The only time I bought a new car in its first model year, I regretted it. It was a 1990 Ford Explorer, and it was a dog. I would rather wait a year or two and allow the problems to be discovered and hopefully fixed. And in medical care it takes even longer to sort out whether "new" really is "improved."

Recognize advertising for what it is: advertising. We've gotten really good at marketing: medical care and laundry detergent can be equally overhyped. But effective marketing doesn't mean effective care. "New" may represent a genuine medical breakthrough—but more often it does not. And there are reasons to be cautious about new drugs, new procedures, and new devices. Each may not really work; each may bring unexpected harm. Given these uncertainties, I would pass on new therapies and stick with the established ones that are known to work.

However, in the case of AIDS in 1990 and metastatic breast cancer, the established therapies were known *not* to work—or, at least, known not to work well. These were tragic situations: deadly diseases affecting young men and women with no good established therapy. Of course there was great enthusiasm to try something new. Yet the only way for medicine to learn that "new" was "improved" for the former—but not for the latter—was to have patients willing to participate in randomized trials.

I hope you never face an analogous situation where new is the only hope, because old offers so little. But if you do, I hope you will be given the option of participating in a randomized trial—and that you give it serious consideration.

Most of medical care, thankfully, is not like this. We have established therapies for many diseases once considered deadly. Moreover, most of medical care is not about acute, life-threatening disease—it's about managing chronic disease (or lowering the risk of disease).

In other words, there is plenty of time. Time to consider options. And should you consider the option of therapy, time to ask about its track record.

If none exists, I'd take the time to find a tried-and-true alternative.

IT'S ALL ABOUT AVOIDING DEATH

Disturbing truth: A fixation on
preventing death diminishes life

"Our new Constitution is now established, and has an
appearance that promises permanency; but in this world
nothing can be said to be certain, except death and taxes."

I'M NOT SURE WHY Franklin equated death with taxes in his 1789 letter to
Jean-Baptiste Leroy. Maybe Ben wrote it immediately after being hit by
lightning. Get real: a number of people seem to be able to avoid paying
taxes, but not one of them will avoid death. Before you start to ponder
whether I have been recently exposed to lightning, let me acknowledge
this chapter title is more than a little imprecise. But then again so is the
language commonly used to promote medical care: it saves lives.

The semantics are relevant here. Saving life and avoiding death are
typically shorthand for far less evocative terms: lengthening life and
delaying death. To be sure, sometimes the language of "saving life" is
warranted: when a young healthy child experiences a life-threatening
problem—such as choking on a piece of hot dog—that is quickly solved
with a definitive, typically simple, medical intervention such as the
Heimlich maneuver. No one would question the "saving life" label here
or the desirability of the intervention. But most of medical care is less
dramatic, and its desirability is more open to question.

Medicine is often described as dealing with life-and-death issues. Occasionally, we are doing just that. But far more often we're dealing less with life and death, more with what kind of life.

I don't look forward to death, nor do I look forward to writing about it. It's an intensely personal issue—one for which I cannot claim any special authority. I don't believe any one doctor, or any one individual, can make that claim. This is value judgment territory: ultimately you have to decide what you value. But I'd be remiss were I to avoid the topic—because a singular focus on avoiding death drives a lot of harmful medical care.

DEATH IS NOT THE ONLY THING THAT MATTERS

Soon after I arrived as a junior faculty member at Dartmouth, I was asked to give a lecture to the medical students. It was nothing special about me, mind you—med schools are always looking for junior faculty to put in front of students.

I was following C. Everett Koop, the former surgeon general and my former boss in the US Public Health Service. Dr. Koop was in the Dartmouth College class of 1937 and had recently returned to teach at the medical school. Because he had said it so often before, I had a pretty good idea of what he was going to say. I even put it on my first slide—which I just had to struggle to open, because old versions of PowerPoint aren't compatible with new ones (which, in my opinion, puts software manufacturers somewhere between device and soap manufacturers). Sorry . . . here's the slide:

There is one thing we all know we can never have too much of, namely, prevention.

—C. EVERETT KOOP, MD

Which was followed by an even simpler slide:

QUESTION AUTHORITY

Dr. Koop's statement was just the kind of dogma that made my blood pressure too high. On first inspection, the statement is apparently reasonable. But on reflection, it is extreme.

I want to be clear, I have a lot of respect for Dr. Koop. It's hard to imagine anyone who could have dealt with the AIDS epidemic better. At the same time, it's hard to imagine anything you can never have too much of. Ice cream? Nope. Exercise? Nope. Sleep? Nope. Beer? Definitely nope; I learned that in high school. And prevention is such a broad term that it could apply to all of medicine. We work to prevent disease, to prevent the complications of disease, and to prevent death.

Never too much? It prompted me to encourage the students to do a thought experiment. I should be clear that what follows is not *my* thought experiment—remember I've never had an original idea in my life. Teachers and researchers always build on the work of others. If it is *your* thought experiment, I apologize for not acknowledging that on the slide:

> *Imagine you discover a tiny blemish on your right fourth toe. Your doctor says it's an exceedingly rare form of cancer. If the toe is removed, you will be cured and will live out a normal life.*
>
> *If not, you will experience a horrible death in six weeks . . .*

"What do you want to do?" I yelled. "Take the toe!" they yelled back. Medical students always appreciate an easy question. So I ramped it up a notch.

> *Imagine you discover a tiny blemish on your right fourth toe. Your doctor says it's an exceedingly rare form of cancer. If the foot is removed, you will be cured and will live out a normal life.*
>
> *If not, you will experience a horrible death in six weeks . . .*

"Take the foot!" they yelled. I ramped it up another notch: *If the leg is amputated below the knee.* And another: an *above* the knee amputation. Now there was less yelling. One more: a hemi-pelvectomy (amputating the leg and one of your hips—with no replacement). Now it was getting quiet.

If you think this is kind of ghoulish, let me remind you it's not *my* thought experiment. But just to show I can get in the spirit of things, I took it to the logical extreme: "Since the pelvis and lower abdomen are not critical to life, how about amputating half your torso?" Cutting you in half—or using more formal surgical nomenclature: a hemi-torsectomy . . .

Never too much? All of a sudden the "horrible death" sounds better than the "horrible treatment"—and the "horrible life."

We tend to think of death—more specifically, avoiding it—as the most important outcome of medicine. It's tempting to think it trumps everything else. But, of course, that's an oversimplification.

WHAT DO PATIENTS WANT?

I have done a fair amount of research over the years and have had the opportunity to serve as a mentor to younger clinicians interested in research. These fellows and junior faculty members may be primary care practitioners or they may be specialists. I like working with the primary care docs because I have a shared understanding of the problems they are interested in; I like working with the specialists because I get to learn about problems I haven't thought much about.

Soon after I joined the medical staff at the White River Junction VA, I was approached by two different specialists who were both interested in the same research question. Gerard was a pulmonologist; Rob was an oncologist. What question do a lung doctor and a cancer doctor have in common? You can guess: it probably has something to do with lung cancer.

I've already argued that lung cancer is, hands down, the most important cancer in the United States. It is responsible for more cancer deaths than any other cancer, more than the next four most-common (colon, breast, pancreas, and prostate) combined. It's even more important in the VA for a simple reason: our patient population includes a lot of smokers. That's why Gerard and Rob were working together a great deal; they were taking care of lung cancer patients in our VA. While most of these patients cannot be helped with surgery, they can be helped with chemotherapy. The benefit of chemotherapy is moderate, however, and it comes at a human cost: more time in the hospital and more time feeling sick—as in fatigue, weakness, nausea, diarrhea, infection, and fever. The question that Gerard and Rob were interested in was, given these trade-offs, what do patients want?

They did structured interviews with patients cared for in a variety of settings—an academic medical center, the VA, and community practice. The eighty-one patients had two things in common: (1) they all had advanced lung cancer and (2) they all had received chemotherapy. That's a great group to talk to. There is nothing for these patients to have to imagine; they knew what it was like to have lung cancer, and they knew what it was like to have chemotherapy.

The structured interviews were designed to assess patient utilities—how individuals value different health-care outcomes. In this case the two outcomes were the length of life and the sickness caused by chemotherapy. The patients were given a series of scenarios where they were asked to choose between accepting chemotherapy or not. What changed in the different scenarios was how much additional life would be gained from accepting chemotherapy. In other words, Gerard and Rob's question was: How long would these patients' lives have to be extended for them to be willing to have chemotherapy again?

A few of the patients would do it again even if chemotherapy only added one week to their life. Others would not do it again even if chemotherapy added two years to their life. This is a key finding: different patients want different things.

What's the actual life-extension benefit of chemotherapy for advanced lung cancer? On average, it's about three months. When given the choice about having chemotherapy or not, only 22 percent of these patients said they would choose chemotherapy to extend their life for three months. In other words, using the best estimate of the effectiveness of treatment in this situation, most patients don't want it.

Why not? Because the treatment is not innocuous, it's hard. These patients understood that in a way none of the rest of us can. And the benefit of treatment is modest. Sure, some might beat the average and get more than three months. But be equally clear, that also implies some get less. Modest, uncertain benefit with certain side effects. Live longer, but spend more of your remaining life in the hospital.

For these patients, at least, it's not all about avoiding death.

MY EXPERIENCE WITH DEATH

Ghoulish thought experiments and utility assessments are scientific tools used to deduce our values about life and death. These values are shaped by personal experience. Because death is such a personal issue, allow me to share mine.

I first saw a dead person at age nineteen as a paramedic in Boulder. A rock climber in Eldorado Canyon had fallen over one hundred feet. My partner and I didn't accept the death; that wasn't our job. We started IVs, placed an endotracheal tube, and did CPR all the way back to the hospital, where the doctors told us to stop. That is what paramedics should do. Our job was to "save lives" and I loved it.

I developed a more nuanced view about death during my first year of medical school. Medical school starts with death—or at least it used to. At the University of Cincinnati, we met our cadaver on day one: a dead human we would share our first year with. The class was gross anatomy—in which the word "gross" refers not to its high school usage but to a macro scale—to distinguish the class from microscopic anatomy (histology). While considerable effort was made to desensitize us to spending so much time with a dead body, there was a concomitant effort to have us recognize the gift that the individual had made. Dissecting a human being is a privilege.

My cadaver was shared with three other students. I remember her well. I particularly remember when my father came to visit her in late November.

My father was a political scientist. The army had taught him Russian during World War II, and during the 1950s he worked for the Central Intelligence Agency. I know that sounds cool, but he wasn't an operative—he was an analyst, charged with dissecting the various Five Year Plans coming out of Moscow. He knew earlier than most that while the Soviet Union had a formidable military, its economy was rotting from the core. He left Langley in 1960 to join the faculty at the University of Colorado, where he taught for the rest of his life.

My father was quite an anachronism in the 1960s—particularly in Boulder, Colorado. If he was on campus, he was in a suit and tie. The shirt was white, the suit was dark gray, and the tie was nondescript. In the winter, he would don an equally nondescript long gray overcoat and a pair of god-awful black rubber galoshes. He topped it off with a leather briefcase and gray fedora. It looked like he had stepped right out of the 1940s and—as my mother repeatedly pointed out—that was because most of his clothes *were* from the 1940s.

Every day, he walked to work. And he walked home for lunch. I've only recently appreciated what a clever strategy that was: without any particular effort, he had hardwired four miles of walking into each day. That's part of my current Five Year Plan.

The walk to campus took him through "The Hill"—a small commercial district adjacent to the university. During the '60s, The Hill was the headquarters for Boulder's counterculture: street people, hippies, freaks, the STP family—and, of course, curious Boulder High School students like me. In fact, I was there twice a day—walking to and from school. It was a quite a scene: music, drugs, and homemade clothing using every color in the rainbow. And my old man would walk through this scene looking like he was headed to Grand Central to catch the 6:05 on the New York, New Haven, and Hartford Railroad.

As my friends pointed out: "He is so far out, he's in."

He was a devoted teacher. His subject matter was timely: US-Soviet relations were a big deal at the time, particularly as they played out in places like Vietnam. A number of my high school classmates went on to have him as a professor in college, and he always received high marks. He cared a great deal about teaching and he was good at it.

But when I got sick as a kid—or had a bloody nose, or managed to hit my face with the back of an ax—it was Mom's problem. It wasn't because my father lacked compassion—quite the opposite, he was the more caring of the two. It was because he lacked competence: he knew nothing about clinical medicine. Mom was a nurse.

So I really looked forward to my father's visit to Cincinnati in the fall of 1977: it was a chance for me to show off. As my daughter would say, it was an opportunity for the student to become the teacher. I knew he wanted to come to our lectures; he always enjoyed watching other professors teach. I asked him if he also wanted to come to gross anatomy lab. He did.

We were in the midst of the best part of gross anatomy at the time— dissecting the chest and abdomen. I say "best" because it is really fascinating to see all those big structures: the heart, the lungs, the liver, the stomach, the spleen, and what seemed like miles and miles of intestine (in fact, closer to twenty-five to thirty feet).

I was surprised how attentive my father was. He seemed to be genuinely interested. It was all new to him. He was a social scientist, not a natural scientist. I was having a great time being the tour guide. We toured the chest cavity, and I explained the mechanics of how a flattened diaphragm created negative pressure, allowing us to breathe. We toured the abdomen. He was impressed by the size of the liver—*Who wouldn't be?*—it's a huge organ. I was on a roll, ready to dive into the detail of the digestive tract. I pointed out that our cadaver was not quite anatomically correct, because she had had a portion of her intestine— her sigmoid colon—surgically removed.

The same operation my father was to have about five weeks later.

My first year of medical school quickly turned into one of the hardest years of my life—and one of the most important.

I went home for a week at Christmas, and my father didn't feel well. He didn't have much energy and was vaguely nauseous and constipated.

He thought he had a "stomach flu"—one that had lasted most of the fall. A few days after I returned to school, Mom took him to the doctor.

He had colon cancer—in his sigmoid colon—and it had spread to multiple places throughout his liver. My father proudly reported on his conversation with the surgeon. He understood what a sigmoid resection was; he had just seen the anatomy. He knew about the liver and how important it was.

He also knew he was about to die. The surgeon said he had about six weeks.

I was taught to avoid giving such precise prognoses. But, then again, there is no disputing that the surgeon was just about right. And please allow me to pass on making a judgment about whether he needed an operation—that was a question Mom asked me repeatedly over the ensuing decades.

She didn't ask it then, however, as she was powering up for a major life event. She was getting up to speed on a then relatively new innovation in medicine—hospice—and was working the phone looking for a physician who was open to what we now would call palliative care. She was also arranging times for each of three boys to spend a weekend alone with their father.

My father was weak when I came home for my long weekend. He was a couple weeks out from the first operation of his life—and his first dose of chemo. He had decided one operation and one chemo dose was enough. Like his father before him, he wanted to die at home. He had accepted death and he wanted to talk about it. He wasn't bitter, quite the opposite. He wanted me to know what a good life he'd had—and how much his sons had contributed to that. And I think he wanted to teach me one last lesson: I need not be scared of death.

My father didn't see death as a final event. He saw it as a transition.

This all makes my father sound so serious. He wasn't. He was actually pretty funny—or at least, he thought he was pretty funny. He was a huge Groucho Marx fan and took me to every Marx Brothers film showing on campus. He penned short playlets making fun of his mother and her sister who lived next door. There was even a mistake-prone physician character (Dr. Wong). He'd read them aloud whenever his two sisters and younger brother got together. They would laugh and laugh. Making fun of one's parents and thinking oneself is funny runs throughout my father's family. It's probably a genetic thing, because my daughter suffers from the same problem. I bet she got it from her paternal grandfather. Thank god it skipped a generation.

A few weeks later my father slipped into a coma. Mom called the three boys back home. She instructed me to bring along whatever classwork I had. Mom was operating at peak proficiency. She had Boulder's new hospice on the case. She had found a young oncologist who understood palliative care—even though he would not have recognized the term. She had their bedroom set up for comfort care and had classical music playing—my father was also a huge fan of Mozart. She was in full nursing mode, giving me instruction on how to change the sheets while my father remained in bed.

Another thing I sure as hell wasn't taught in medical school.

During the next ten days, my brothers and I spent a lot of time in that bed—next to our father. It was very peaceful: we would read while our father was comfortably resting and listening to Mozart. I was reading neuroanatomy—what a colossal waste of time. Although my father couldn't say anything, I know he would have been amused. He had learned enough about medical school during his visit to wonder about the utility of some of the medical curriculum: too much content, too many alleged "facts," and not enough on the process of critical thinking. We're still working on that. Course corrections take time.

My father's siblings arrived. There was great sadness and crying, of course. But there was also laughing. The oncologist stopped by—and not just to see my father. He knew he was treating an entire family. And he took extra time with me: he clearly recognized I was receiving an education in something much more important than neuroanatomy. He was modeling something more than using oral morphine for pain or atropine to dry secretions so patients breathe easier; he was modeling how to guide families through a profound life event: death.

After about ten days of being in a coma, my father died. He died in his own bed—surrounded by his wife, his three children, and his three siblings.

And thirty-six years later, I'm writing this at my father's desk—with his briefcase next to me. Maybe my father is right: death is just a transition.

DEATH IN AMERICA

If the surveys are right, this is the way most Americans would like to die. In their own home. In the presence of loved ones. No sound of oxygen flowing, suction equipment, intravenous pumps, monitoring devices—or their alarms. No frenetic activity of medical professionals.

Peacefully. It's certainly the way I'd like to die.

But that's not necessarily what happens. The most common place for Americans to die is still in the hospital. A hospital is not a peaceful place. The prevailing paradigm in the hospital is intervention, not comfort. And it is not simply due to the doctors. If you are in the hospital, it is a safe bet that your insurer will want evidence that you need to be there, that something is being done to you—something that couldn't be done somewhere else.

And a standard hospital room is positively bucolic compared to the intensive care unit. ICUs are busy, noisy, frenetic, and frightening places. There are lots of monitoring devices, which detect lots of abnormalities, which leads to lots of uncomfortable procedures. The ICU is not a good place to die.

My colleagues at the *Dartmouth Atlas of Health Care* have been studying end-of-life care for years. There is some good news: the proportion of patients dying in the hospital is falling. Some of this, however, may reflect patients being discharged to nursing homes immediately prior to death. Here's the bad news: patients are increasingly spending part of the last six months of their life in an ICU.

Furthermore, a startling number of doctors can be involved with care at the end of life. One-third of Medicare patients cared for by

"America's Best Hospitals" (as designated by *US News & World Report*) were seen by ten or more physicians during their last six months of life. That's right, ten or more. It's hard to imagine how that can ever be good. These may be our best hospitals, but they are certainly not our best deaths.

Why is American medical care so intensive at the end of life? A big part of the story is the assumption that it is all about avoiding death. Do everything possible.

Doctors assume it's what the patients want. "Saving lives" is our default mode—and, just like the paramedics, for good reason. Patients assume it's what their family wants (or worse, what their doctor wants). Families assume it's what the patient would want (or worse, choose to assume it as a way to demonstrate how much they care.) It's hard to move out of the default mode. It's hard not to do everything possible.

I have witnessed numerous deaths since my father died. Each was guided, however, by that experience. I wanted patients and their families to understand the tension between medical care directed to prolong life and medical care directed to provide comfort—that it is hard for us to make people comfortable while we are doing things to them. I wanted patients to know that there was no single right answer—that they had choices about how to approach death.

I sure knew what Mom wanted. She had thirty-two years to express her preferences following my father's death (not that they weren't obvious, recall she was president of the Hemlock Society...). Other than choosing to have knee replacements, she was a nurse who wanted to stay out of the hospital. She left Boulder in 2002 to move back to her hometown—New Haven, Connecticut—to join a life care retirement community. A few years later she had an ill-defined "spell and fall" that landed her in the hospital where she trained, Yale-New Haven. I arrived a few hours later and told the doctors a little about Mom. They were happy not to pursue a definitive diagnosis; Mom was relieved to go home. And my wife had the foresight to recognize it was time for me to move Mom closer to our home.

Mom never went into the hospital again. There were a couple of times she could have, but I was in a good position to express her strong preferences. She wasn't able to die at home, but in 2010 she was able to die in a quiet room without any frenetic activity of medical professionals. I was there, but not professionally or frenetically, I was in bed beside her. Her siblings couldn't be there—they had died years before. Her other boys were en route (either I was a little slow in calling or Mom jumped the gun—since I'm still around, let's blame her).

A few hours later, my brothers and I gathered around our mother, had a beer, and honored her life. We spent the weekend together: telling stories, reliving childhood memories, and making fun of our parents. Both of my parents would have liked that.

I know more could have been done for—or should I say "to"?—both my father and mother. Since they both undoubtedly had developed pneumonia, both could have lived longer had they had antibiotics and aggressive respiratory care. Since they had both stopped drinking and eating, both could have lived longer had they had intravenous fluids and tube feedings. Much more could have been done to prolong their lives. But it wasn't. We didn't do everything possible.

This course of action wasn't chosen to save money. It was chosen because that is what they wanted. My parents did not have a death wish; they wished to avoid having their deaths medicalized. They viewed that as a fate worse than death: sterile, isolating, and even inhumane.

How do I know? I never saw a living will—although knowing my mother I wouldn't be surprised if she had completed three or four of them over the years. I knew because both my parents spoke directly to their children about death and how they wanted to approach it. I could also see that their lives had not been dominated by efforts to avoid death.

AVOIDING DEATH AT THE PRIME OF LIFE

Until now, I have been considering the desirability of efforts to extend life as individuals approach the time of death. There have been concerns about the role of medical care in death and dying for decades. Questions like "Do you want chemotherapy for advanced lung cancer?" or "If death is near, do you want (pick one) antibiotics, hydration, tube feeding?" are increasingly routine. We have become more sensitized that efforts to avoid death may not make sense at the end of life.

But certainly they make sense in the prime of life. We can never have too much of that kind of prevention, right? Attempting to lower the risk of death (lengthen life) for individuals in the prime of life is a big part of medical care. It often rests on the assumption that it is all that patients care about.

Once again, working with specialists opened my eyes to an issue I hadn't thought much about. For specialized surgical procedures, there is a so-called volume-outcome relationship. The empirical finding is straightforward: hospitals and surgeons who perform an operation frequently (that is, have higher volumes) tend to obtain more favorable results (that is, have better outcomes) than those who perform an operation less frequently. Makes sense—it's simply a variant of the learning curve phenomenon.

The finding that higher volumes are associated with better outcomes—specifically lower operative mortality rates—serves as a major rationale for the regionalization of specialized surgical procedures. The idea is simple: concentrate complex procedures in high-volume centers with high-volume surgeons—so-called "Centers of Excellence"—and fewer patients will die from their operation.

But one of my surgical fellows had the audacity to ask the question: Is that what patients want? I love questions like that. The volume-outcome field had been humming along nicely, showing lower operative mortality rates in high-volume centers and suggesting that procedures be regionalized—all assuming that patients only cared about one thing: avoiding death.

Full disclosure: this surgeon worked for a low-volume hospital—as did I. We worked for the White River Junction VA, a small hospital (currently listed as having seventy-four beds) serving veterans in two predominantly rural states (Vermont and New Hampshire). Sam and I knew two things: (1) in our case regionalization meant Boston and (2) for many of our patients, despite being Boston sports fans, that city was not a desirable destination.

It's not about Boston; it's about how many rural Americans feel about big metropolitan areas: too much traffic, too noisy, too fast-paced—and too far from friends and family. But these aren't patients at the end of life; these are patients considering a surgical procedure. Certainly they'd be willing to go elsewhere to lower their risk of operative death, right?

You never know till you ask.

Sam decided to interview one hundred consecutive patients who were scheduled for elective surgery. That's a good group to talk to: for these individuals, surgery is not some hypothetical possibility; it is something they have thought about carefully and have consented to. The interview was carefully structured: all the patients were directed to consider the same major operation—a big operation, one with a substantial risk of operative death. In the interview scenario the risk of death was 3 percent at the regional hospital, a hospital that was a four-hour drive away (Boston is a little closer to us than that, unless you are trying to get there during rush hour).

The patients were then told the risk of death at the local hospital. At first, they were told it was also 3 percent. Now came the question: Where would you want to have the surgery? All one hundred patients would choose to have their surgery done locally. That's not surprising: it's all tied up—regional 3 percent versus local 3 percent—and local is closer to home.

In the second iteration, the risk of death in the local hospital was raised to 4 percent. Now it's regional 3 percent versus local 4 percent. Again the question: Where would you want to have the surgery?

Three-quarters still wanted to be treated locally—despite the one-third higher risk of death.

Finally, the risk of death was doubled for the local hospital: regional 3 percent versus local 6 percent. Yet, just under half (45 percent) still wanted to be treated locally—despite the doubling in their risk of death.

Once again, different patients want different things. But, even in the prime of life, it's not simply about avoiding death. It's also about being in familiar surroundings—and being close to family and friends.

ANTICIPATORY MEDICINE

Of course, there's more to life than trying to avoid death. If we were just trying to avoid death we'd still be driving 55 mph on the interstate. Endurance cyclists would get off the road and spin in the gym. No one would play football; no one would ride in the rodeo. Kayakers would avoid rapids; skiers would stay in bounds. And I wouldn't hike by myself (pretty extreme, huh?).

Why don't we always "play it safe"? It's because we make a judgment: the risk of death from these activities is relatively small, while their value is relatively large. A little extra risk of death; a lot of extra value. Little harm, lots of benefits—so we do it.

There is a similar judgment to be made about medical care—but now the benefit is about reducing the risk of death. In the case of medical care for acute symptomatic disease, there's not only the potential to ward off an impending death, there is also the potential of enabling you to feel better now. In other words, the benefits typically overwhelm the harms.

But the balance is much finer for medical care for the well—particularly efforts to influence the timing and cause of death for those in the prime of life. This is anticipatory medicine: the attempt to anticipate what will go wrong in the future and to address it now. It is a tricky calculus.

The benefit—to the extent it exists—is the potential to lengthen life in the distant future. There are no symptoms to fix—remember it's hard to make a well person feel better. But we can make you worse: make you more anxious about life, add a lot of hassle to an already complex life (appointments to make, phone calls, scripts to fill, insurance forms to fill out), and even cause physical harm (medication side effects, surgical complications, and even death).

Before you sign on to this deal you want to know how big the benefit is, how certain it is, and what harms you might be willing to experience trying to get it.

Here's how I think about it as I approach age sixty. First, there are some things I don't have to anticipate: I am acutely aware that I am aging. My memory isn't what it used to be. My urinary tract doesn't drain the way it used to. I have an increasing number of muscular-skeletal problems: my back regularly goes into spasm when I bend over in the morning, I get shooting pains in my wrist at night, and some muscle in my groin occasionally catches and spasms when I'm walking. Add to that, my memory isn't what it used to be . . .

So without having to anticipate anything, we could have a lengthy debate about whether I really am well. While I can imagine a number of things I could offer a patient such as myself, I have chosen not to pursue diagnostic testing. The likelihood of adding some useful information from testing is remarkably low. The likelihood of adding some distracting information, on the other hand, is quite high. A similar situation exists for the treatments that might be plausibly initiated. The likelihood that one would help a great deal is low (because none of these problems are that bothersome—and because our interventions for them are pretty pathetic), while the likelihood that one might cause new problems is reasonably high.

If the problems get worse, I'll happily reconsider this decision. And I can anticipate that some of these problems will likely get worse—or that new ones will crop up—as I get older.

I know death is in my future.

A TRAGEDY OR A BLESSING?

I also know death isn't always a bad thing. There are different types of death. My father died of metastatic colon cancer at age sixty; my mother died of dementia as she approached age ninety. There is absolutely no question: Mom's death was a good thing. It was a blessing. She wished it would have come earlier. She wasn't depressed; she just didn't want to live too long. But she did.

Mom would have described my father's death as a tragedy—as it was the most painful loss of her life. But I don't believe my father would characterize his death that way. He lived six years longer than his father, he had a chance to see his three children launched—he recognized he had had a good life. His death was sad, but not a tragedy. He would have reserved that word for the death of one of his children—or anyone in that age group at the time.

Time marches on. Now the word *tragedy* would be appropriate for another generation: my daughter's. The generation who otherwise have their whole lives before them, like a high school student killed in a horrible car accident or a young mother who dies from metastatic breast cancer. Here is where medical care is most important—if it can avert tragedy. In fact, one of medicine's biggest success stories is that breast cancer deaths in women under forty have been cut almost in half. And this is not about screening—this age group is rarely screened; it's about better treatment. That's great news.

I'm no longer a tragedy candidate. To the extent that I can choose the circumstances of my death, it would be between a sad one and a blessing. I don't want my father's death, but I don't want my mother's either. And I probably won't get to choose anyway. So how much time and effort—physical, emotional, monetary—do I want to devote to fiddling around with this question when I've got a life to live now?

Do I want to enroll in anticipatory medicine?

I know medical care has some capacity—albeit limited—to influence my cause of death. I'm almost certainly at lower than average risk for a heart disease death. So if there is a disease with my name on it, it's cancer. And if there is a cancer with my name on it, given my professional work, it's prostate cancer. A number of urologists might think that would be particularly fitting. I'm kidding, they are generally good people. Nor do I think there are any mammographers who would like to see me die from breast cancer (it can happen to men)—although a couple have e-mailed my dean saying that I should be fired, honestly.

I know I could develop metastatic prostate cancer and die from it. I know taking my prostate out would reduce (but not eliminate) my chance of this outcome. I believe PSA screening can also reduce this chance to a much smaller degree—but largely because it leads to so many prostatectomies. I simply don't want that degree of intervention, that much harm to possibly change something that could happen, but much more likely won't. That's why I don't get screened for prostate cancer.

Not surprisingly, the cancer I've thought most about getting is colon cancer. When my older brothers turned fifty, they asked me whether I thought they should get a colonoscopy. Given our father's history, I said yes. When I turned fifty, I got one. That's not news; it was in the *New York Times* in 2004 (not a headline mind you, just in an interview about my first book, *Should I Be Tested for Cancer? Maybe Not and Here's Why*).

All three of us had normal findings. That says something to me: my father's colon cancer, like most colon cancer, was likely a sporadic cancer—simply put: it was bad luck. Given our colonoscopy findings, the best bet now is that my brothers and I are not at elevated risk but at average risk for colon cancer—or, arguably, below average, given that no polyps were found.

One more thing: the average risk of developing colon cancer is going down. Colon cancer incidence has fallen almost 40 percent since my father died. And don't make the mistake of thinking this is all the result of screening—the incidence started falling long before screening became commonplace. Something else is going on, something good. If you don't think something good can happen without medical care, consider this: since the 1950s, stomach cancer has virtually disappeared—its incidence has fallen 80 percent—and no one is screening for it.

I've been invited back for a colonoscopy a number of times since then—I must have been an exemplary patient. In fact, I just got an invitation in the mail yesterday (you just can't make this stuff up). Haven't taken them up on any of the invitations, not sure I ever will (if I do one more, it will definitely be my last).

You might think that's because I found my colonoscopy unpleasant. Quite the opposite. I actually looked forward to it. Not only had I told my brothers to get one, I had referred many patients to get the procedure. I thought it was a good time for me to experience being a patient.

I was bound and determined to have a "good prep"—to have my colon totally clear of stool—to ensure that my gastroenterologist could see well. I was amazed how much diarrhea the gallon of "Go Lyte" caused and how little it bothered me (most diarrheas make you feel weak from dehydration). It's amazing stuff.

And the procedure itself was even better. My same-day surgery nurse was a next-door neighbor—our daughters played basketball together for a decade. My gastroenterologist was a former fellow—someone whom I had played basketball with (even though I didn't belong on the same court). He gave me some great drugs (the same he gives all patients): it didn't hurt a bit. I felt great and was wide awake. I was even able to watch the whole thing on TV—in real time.

Truth is, I thoroughly enjoyed it. But I'm a doctor. Simply having the experience of being a patient was novel. Even more fascinating was the experience of seeing one's own anatomy: the inside of the colon. Watching the colonoscope make it around the corners—the splenic and hepatic flexures—was particularly cool.

So why am I not sure I'll ever do it again? I know I could still die from colon cancer, but how much do I want to concern myself with a relatively rare cause of death? The truth is that the procedure has, at best, a very tiny chance of influencing my longevity. Furthermore, I'm not even sure what direction I want my longevity to go. By lowering my risk of colon cancer death, might I be raising my chance of dying of dementia—after years of requiring assistance with the activities of daily living?

And just because I'm not enthusiastic about further colon cancer screening doesn't mean I'm closed to any preventive intervention. I'm on a blood pressure medicine now. Why? Not because I am sure I want to live longer but because I am sure I would like to try to avoid having a stroke. There's no one right approach to anticipatory medicine *because there's no one right approach to life and death.* It's personal.

PRESCRIPTION: STRIVE TO LIVE LIFE, NOT AVOID DEATH

We've been taught to fear death—or view it as some sort of failure. I fear medical care has had some role in this, as it often proceeds as if extending life is the only goal. It's a paradigm based on a number of assumptions that you may want to question.

First, *is extending life always a desirable goal?* It's easy for me to imagine scenarios for which the answer is no: I'm in pain, in a long-term care facility, but I'm not sure where—nor am I sure who my wife and daughter are. No, at that point, I don't want to be treated for pneumonia, have my blood pressure lowered (or raised), or be screened for cancer.

Although it is easier to understand why efforts to extend life might not be desirable at the end of life, it's tougher in the middle of life. For me, the effort feels like gambling: trading off chances of living a life that is too short against those of a life too long. And the effort to fiddle around with those chances feels like a distraction from living life. But that's just me. I leave it to you to consider whether extending life is always a desirable goal for you.

Second, *is extending life always an achievable goal?* Will medical care always lengthen life? No cancer screening test in an average risk population has ever been shown to do that. I'm not saying that screening might not have some effect on overall mortality, just that it's such a small effect that it's virtually impossible for us to measure. This serves as a distinct contrast to intervention for acute illness or injury, where treatment is regularly shown to prolong life. If life extension is a desirable outcome for you, sign on to acute care medicine. Be more circumspect about the anticipatory flavor.

We also know that some people do better with less focus on extending life. A study of 151 patients with advanced lung cancer randomized patients to receive either life-extending care or palliative care—care directed not to extending their life, but to addressing their symptoms and the stress of terminal illness. The palliative care group had less aggressive medical care: less time in the hospital, fewer trips to the emergency room, less likely to be given chemotherapy as they neared death. And they lived, on average, almost three months longer.

Sometimes we can try too hard to extend life—and end up shortening it. Many doctors have had the experience of withdrawing life-extending care in the hospital, only to see their patient's condition improve. A similar phenomenon exists in the outpatient world. Many frail elderly patients have accumulated multiple medications from various doctors intended to extend life. Sometimes these patients get frustrated, stop all their medications—and do much better. I'm not advocating this course of action, but I am a big fan of rule five in Dr. Sidney Wolfe's "Ten Rules for Safer Drug Use": "Stopping a Drug Is as Important as Starting It."

Finally, *is extending life the only goal of life?* The paradigm of extending life frequently incorporates a heroic assumption: nothing else matters. If extending life is both desirable and achievable, it should be pursued—regardless of the human cost.

If mammography "saves lives"—however few and however uncertain—should we instruct all women to do it despite the harm of overdiagnosis and the fact that it has made breast cancer scares a rite of passage for middle-aged American women?

Never too much? Nothing else matters when the effort is to save a life? Can I interest you in a hemi-torsectomy? Sorry if that's too ghoulish. How about frequent bloody noses that stain your shirts, ties, and sheets? Sorry if that's too gross (high school usage). Here's the real question: Why aren't you driving 55?

Probably because other things do matter. Your life is not all about avoiding death. Consider whether you want your medical care to reflect that. When it comes to anticipatory medicine, you need to make your own decision about what else matters to you. But if becoming medicalized while you feel well is not high on your list, you need to say so.

Embrace life. And don't dwell on death—recognize that it's part of life.

CONCLUSION

Seeking medical care is *not* the most important thing you can do for your health

OF COURSE, THERE ARE more than just seven assumptions that drive too much medical care. I just liked the way the number seven sounded (don't ask me why, four is really my favorite digit). You should know, however, I did consider some others:

Specialists are always better

Disturbing truth: Specialty care is typically more invasive and chaotic and can miss the forest for the trees.

But I didn't want to anger more than half my colleagues—most American physicians are specialists.

Doctors always know what they are doing

Disturbing truth: Doctors are human, and the science of medical care is imperfect and will always be.

But I didn't want to anger my remaining colleagues. Plus, since you've gotten this far, you can see we've already touched on this issue.

■ ■ ■

SO, NO MORE ASSUMPTIONS. Books have to end sometime—and I've got to get back to work anyway. But I should conclude with some consideration of the role of medical care in health, particularly in a book titled *Less Medicine, More Health*. And that requires some consideration of what constitutes health.

WHAT IS HEALTH?

In 1895, the State of Wyoming "discovered" several large hot springs flowing into the Bighorn River just north of the Wind River Canyon. Governor William Richards recommended that the 3rd Wyoming Legislature *"invite the attention of Congress"* to bequeath these springs to the state. He noted that doing so would be *"a boon to suffering humanity"* and that among the *"average attendance of more than 100 people daily . . . no patient failed of being materially benefitted."*

A year later, Shoshone chief Washakie entered into an agreement with the US government to sell a ten-mile square of land surrounding the Big Horn Hot Springs with the provision that a portion should be forever reserved for the use and benefit of the public. It's been called "The Gift of the Waters," although it's not clear Chief Washakie was in much of a position to pursue an alternative strategy. The following year the springs were transferred to the state.

And more than a century later the State of Wyoming still maintains a bathhouse that is free to all. If you are ever in the Bighorn Basin, I suggest you stop by to be materially benefited. There's nothing like a good soak to make you feel better.

Who would have thought the state of Wyoming would have been an early adopter of a broader view of health?

In 1947, the World Health Organization formulated a definition of health:

Health is a state of complete physical, mental and social well-being and not merely the absence of disease or infirmity.

Wow. As Richard Smith, a former editor of the *British Medical Journal*, once quipped, it's a definition that *"would leave most of us unhealthy most of the time."* Complete physical, mental, and social well-being is certainly a state I can only approach transiently when soaking in a hot spring. Plus I need a cold beer—which is not allowed at the state baths.

The same journal encouraged a conversation and a conference about the definition of health. In 2011, they came up with this:

> the ability to adapt and self manage in the face of social, physical, and emotional challenges

The ability to adapt to changing circumstances is an important component of health. In a word, it's about resilience: after something bad happens—the ability to become strong, healthy, or successful again.

But you can be resilient and die tomorrow. If this is the result of acute lead toxicity or a gunshot wound, most would acknowledge that the individual was probably not in a healthy environment. Something about longevity—with a particular focus on reducing premature deaths—is clearly relevant in a definition of health.

And you can be resilient and still feel crummy. Certainly "feeling good" oughta be in there somewhere—although to appear in publications of the World Health Organization or the British Medical Association, it might need to be stated more formally.

There's no one right definition of health. But there are wrong ones.

My medical training never included a formal definition of health. Why would it? But we did have an operational definition: We say you are healthy if we can't find anything wrong with you. It's nothing about your ability to adapt to adversity, how long you'll live, or how you feel. That stuff is too hard to measure. Our convention has been to define health as the absence of abnormality.

That is a wrong definition. As you are now aware, today we doctors can find abnormalities in virtually everyone. This is the result of three factors: (1) the increasing ability of our diagnostic technologies to detect minute perturbations in our anatomy, physiology, biochemistry, and genome; (2) our overly narrow definitions of what constitutes normal; and (3) our increasing tendency to look hard to see if we can't find something wrong.

Health is something about a physical state, but it is also something about a state of mind.

THE DETERMINANTS OF HEALTH

Now that we've cleared that up, let's move on to my public health training. One of the first concepts taught to students upon entering a school of public health is the determinants of health—the variety of factors that determine health. I was one of the physicians in the back of the room whose eyes were glazing over. Had I been paying attention, I might have asked exactly what the determinants were determining.

Although the determinants of health are variably enumerated, they are consistently numerous. And, honestly, I don't think it matters exactly how you define health: however you choose to define it, there are bound to be multiple determinants of it. The World Health Organization, for example, currently lists ten determinants of health: income and social status, education, physical environment, employment and working conditions, social support networks, culture, genetics, personal behavior and coping skills, health services, and gender.

The general point is well taken: medical care is only one of multiple determinants of health. It's an important point. Let's consider the other nine, starting with the things you are stuck with (our jargon would be "not modifiable").

1. *Gender.* Not much to say here, except, *"Guys, to the extent health is about longevity, you lose."*
2. *Genetics.* Your genes are basically hard-wired, unless you want to consider gene therapy. Which I suggest you don't—unless you have a severe genetic disorder, understand that many attempts have failed, and are in a clinical trial. For most of us, genetic

information is something you (and your doctor) take as a given and have to choose whether or not to react to. And the kind of genetic information you are most likely to want to react to is contained in the oldest genetic test of all: your family history.

OK. With this pair of determinants, you are stuck with the cards you are dealt. Let's move on to those that are, at least, potentially modifiable.

3. *Income and social status.* This is a powerful determinant of health. The classic evidence for it is the Whitehall Study of the 1970s, which delineated the health status of British civil servants. The higher the grade level of employment (more income, more social status), the better the physical and mental health—and the lower the mortality. No surprise here. The question of how much we want to modify this determinant of health is a question for public policy everywhere, particularly in a time of widening income disparity.

4. *Education.* Of course, I think education is an important determinant of health. But then again I'm an educator. In fact, the word *doctor* implies being a teacher. But let's be clear, educational attainment is inexorably linked to income and social status. And if forced to choose between being highly educated with low income/low social status versus being poorly educated with high income/high social status, most of us would choose the latter. We should be careful not to overweight the value of education—just as we should not overweight the value of medical care.

5. *Employment and working conditions.* It's getting messier. Now we've got three things inexorably linked together: income/social status, education, and employment. Having a decent paying job (income) and doing work that is valued (status) and safe (working conditions) undoubtedly do contribute to health. It is probably all wrapped up in the phrase "good job," which politicians and policymakers are rightfully concerned about. James Carville was right: "It's the economy, stupid."

6. *Physical environment.* Sounds like we're back to the issue of lead. But I bet when the World Health Organization constructed their list, their primary interest was in a different variable: access to clean water. Keeping water clean requires basic sanitation, the safe disposal of human urine and feces. It was a critical step in reducing the transmission of a variety of infectious diseases. Don't get me wrong, clean air is important too—it was good to get the lead out.

7. *Social support networks.* Isolation is typically not good for health. It is good to get beyond oneself. We all like being cared for. And caring for friends, families, and communities offers its own rewards.

8. *Culture.* I don't know much about culture (or, if you're really from Boston, "kultcha"). I don't got any anyway. It seems a safe bet, however, that how important culture is to health depends on how broadly one defines the term. It's certainly less about a culture of arts, more about a culture of behaviors. I suspect the hunting culture is good for health. It combines physical activity, respect for the land and the animals, and purpose: putting food on the table. I'm less sanguine about a gun culture. I am sure that if a culture becomes hell-bent on shooting at each other, it won't be good for the public's health.

And, finally, on to the last determinant—the most modifiable—and the one you are most likely to hear about from your doctor.

9. *Personal Behavior.* This is the stuff I keep reminding you that your grandmother might have told you when you were young: get plenty of sleep, eat your fruits and vegetables, go play outside—and don't start smoking. Given that it roughly doubles the overall rate of death (the combination of deaths from lung cancer, heart disease, and all other causes), cigarette smoking tops the list of personal behaviors relevant to health. Since I have already beaten that into the ground, let's move on to the next most relevant personal behaviors: diet and exercise.

Diet and exercise . . . it sounds so unappealing. The word *diet* feels like a chemistry lab: add two milliliters of this to four grams of that. And the word *exercise* evokes the image of a treadmill: working hard, not getting anywhere. But it doesn't have to be that way. Allow me to nominate some alternative words:

FOOD AND MOVEMENT

That's better. Before I go further, I should acknowledge one thing: it is easier for medical care to meet the gold standard of evidence than it is for the other determinants of health. In other words, while we can randomize patients to receive drugs and procedures, we can't randomize them to be rich or poor, to have social supports or not, or to eat Brussels sprouts or Cheetos. With that proviso, let's explore what I think is an emerging consensus about food and movement.

Eating shouldn't be a chemistry lab; just try to get most of your calories from plants. Fruits, vegetables, whole grains, and legumes not only contain a lot of nutrients; they contain a lot of fiber. Filling, but not calorie-dense (*fills you up, not out*). The fruit and vegetable choices available to most of us, regardless of the season, are truly remarkable (as are the choices made by so many grocers to have us walk through their produce section first, so I end up crushing the tomatoes with my beer). Throw in the whole grains and legumes that have been the world's primary calorie source for thousands of years: wheat, corn, barley, rice, beans, lentils, and potatoes (I know it's a root vegetable). I must confess I made fun of the quinoa and soybean crowd in high school, but now we know they were probably on the right track.

This doesn't mean I don't eat meat—in fact, when I have a steak I want to have some real fat on it. And I particularly like meats associated with colon cancer—sausage and salami—and happily ignore the tiny double-digit percentage increase in my risk (as suggested in chapter 1). All I've done is to move away from making meat the centerpiece of the daily menu. And I still throw down the occasional bag of nonfood; I'm quite partial to Cheetos. The key is moderation.

Movement doesn't have to be a physiology lab. My father didn't walk to work to hit a target heart rate—or to get real time physiologic feedback from a muscle oxygen monitor. He walked because he enjoyed it. The standard rationale for regular physical activity is for cardiovascular health, but it is equally important for mental health. The reason to be active is less to avoid a heart attack in the future and more to sleep better, think better, and feel better now.

And it's not all about the heart anyway. One of the reasons I don't like the word "exercise" is that we typically equate it with cardiovascular activity: raising your heart rate, building up heat, and getting short of breath. Don't get me wrong—that's important, but there are other elements to movement that you won't get on a treadmill: range of motion, flexibility, and balance. It's not rocket science. If you want to maintain a range of motion, you must regularly assume a range of positions. It can be as simple as cleaning the house *(forgive me guys)*. And if you want to maintain your balance, you must regularly be in the position to lose your balance. I don't care if you do yoga, Pilates, or Aqua-motion or just walk on uneven surfaces that are occasionally unstable—like the snowy/slushy/icy/poorly shoveled walkways found in so many urban areas this past winter.

Dr. Mike Evans sums up our need for movement in a video titled *Let's Make Our Day Harder*. It's right on, except the title. Once you get moving, I'm confident you'll come to like it, so it becomes "Let's make our day more enjoyable."

OTHER DETERMINANTS OF HEALTH

Even with this expansive list, the World Health Organization almost certainly failed to enumerate all the determinants of health. Many would argue that "purpose" needs to be on the list. To be sure, it's a broad category: caring for children, grandchildren, parents, and grandparents gives people a sense of purpose. And it doesn't have to involve family—simply caring for others can provide a sense of purpose. Ironically, there is some evidence that providing social support is more important to health than receiving it. It might not even have to involve humans—caring for God, animals, plants, or the land itself can give people purpose. The central ingredient is caring about something, having some reason to live.

My brother Jim would make another nomination: having fun. I'll second it. Think about what fun means: something enjoyable or amusing. Something that makes you cheerful or light-hearted, something that makes you feel better now. Joy and laughter are things we typically associate with children at play—something we can forget to do as adults. Anyone up for a snowball fight?

One more determinant to put on the list: luck. Sorry, this one is nonmodifiable. No matter how many determinants of health we throw in the mix, we will never be able to perfectly predict who will experience good health. Some of it is simply luck. Accidents are called that for a reason; any one of us can draw the bad card of an aggressive cancer. Good people—doing all the right things—still get sick. It's tempting to want to find something—or someone—to blame. Too often the blame is placed on the patient. It's important to acknowledge the role of chance in health.

MODERATING MEDICINE

"Seek moderation in all things" is nearly the only thing I know about Aristotle. Honestly, I was first exposed to it in a Dave Berg comic in *Mad* magazine. Yet it is an idea that has stuck with me as being extremely relevant to health.

The determinants of health are not presented as a list of things to do: "I must eat quinoa," "I must do Pilates," "I must have fun" (that only makes it harder to have fun, anyway).

Don't try to do everything right—part of moderation is not getting too wrapped up in it. While it is not healthy to ignore one's health, it also is not healthy to obsess about it. Pursuing health requires, ironically, not paying too much attention to it.

Instead I share the determinants of health to convey a central idea: human health is the product of a variety of factors. Medical care is just one of them—and thus, by itself, a relatively weak determinant of health.

Medical care can be extremely valuable. But that does not imply it is routinely valuable. Because of the dramatic impact medical care can have on human health, it is tempting to think that seeking it is the most important thing you can do for your health. That exaggerates the importance of medical care: doctors don't reliably make people feel more resilient (sadly, in the case of those who are well, often the reverse), we can't make everybody feel good, and we are not the arbitrator of who lives or dies. The reality is more nuanced: medical care is most likely to be important when you are acutely sick or injured—while staying well is a different ball game.

To understand the value of moderation in medical care, you need to understand that it too follows a U-shaped curve. Just as you can have a blood pressure or blood sugar that is too low, you can have too little medical care. And just as you can have a blood pressure or blood sugar that is too high, you can have too much medical care. Because the problem of too much is so much less familiar than the problem of too little, I have focused on the harms of excessive medical care. At the same time, I hope I have conveyed a balanced view.

My motivation for writing this book rests on a firm belief: if the American public knew the full story about the benefits, harms, and uncertainties of medical care, many would choose to have less. Not less care, less medicine—meaning the interventions of testing, medication, procedures, surgeries, and devices. Obviously, I haven't given you the whole story here. That would take multiple volumes, because there are so many dimensions to medicine. And there would be a lot of missing pages, because there is much we do not know.

But I hope that I have given you some sense of the landscape. How medical excess can be harmful is probably most familiar at the end of life. Here it is easy to see how aggressive intervention in the dying is not only futile, but inhumane.

Medical excess is equally prevalent, however, at the other extreme of health: care for the well. The resulting harms are less familiar. Efforts to anticipate what might go wrong—but has not—are fraught with uncertainty, as is the question of what to do about it. Any plausible benefit occurs in the future, as it is hard for doctors to make the well feel any better now. Unfortunately, it is less hard for us to make them feel worse.

Caring for the well and those at the end of life are the two settings in which moderation is most called for. They are also the settings in which you are best positioned to influence your care.

Acute care medicine is different. The complex interplay of all the determinants of health has now played out. There's no need to anticipate: genetic factors, environmental factors, and the role of chance have combined to produce an obvious problem.

Nevertheless, moderation is still relevant to the sick. Some problems are better managed than solved. Less data can hasten recovery. Inaction can allow healing. And the old standby may be better than the next big thing. Increasingly physicians understand these things; let yours know that you do too.

ACKNOWLEDGMENTS

MAYBE IT GOES WITHOUT SAYING: I am responsible for all the words in this book. But I'm certainly not responsible for all the ideas. There are many doctors who worry about the excesses of medical care—and many who have influenced my thinking.

Two stand out. Jack Wennberg had a lot to do with my coming to Dartmouth and creating a research environment that encouraged the questioning of established medical practices. More importantly, he helped me recognize that the most fundamental medical question was not *"How much does it cost?"* but *"Does it really help people?"* Bill Black, whom I met soon after arriving at Dartmouth, sensitized me to the ambiguities of diagnosis: that patients don't simply either "have" or "not have" a diagnosis, but instead there is a substantial spectrum of gray in between. More importantly, he helped me understand how these ambiguities could influence our perceptions of both how much disease there is and whether our interventions help.

Having access to ideas is one thing—getting them down on paper is another. Truth is, I find writing to be hard work (I don't even like writing the acknowledgments section). However, writing mentors early in my career—Eric Larson, Fred Connell, Peter Mogielnicki, and my brother Pete—did teach me one thing: writing is a social exercise, not something to be done alone. This book has been influenced by a number of what I call "internal reviewers"—individuals who have read and commented on various sections or chapters—who are listed below. While they cannot be held responsible for the words, I am indebted for their critique.

I also appreciate the help of both my brothers—who each reviewed a chapter—for bringing their distinct perspectives to bear. My wife, on the other hand, was prevailed upon to read the whole thing. And more than once. Linda's comments—and support—proved invaluable.

—H. Gilbert Welch
Thetford, Vermont

INTERNAL REVIEWERS

Bruce Andrus, MD (cardiology), Dartmouth-Hitchcock Medical Center

Kyle Barrus (undergraduate), Montana State University

Wylie Burke, MD (genetics), University of Washington

Ira Byock, MD (palliative care), Missoula, Montana

Richard Deyo, MD, MPH (family medicine), Oregon Health Sciences University

Sam Finlayson, MD (general surgery), University of Utah

Sara Graves, MD (orthopedics), Dartmouth-Hitchcock Medical Center

David Grossman, MD (pediatrics), Group Health Cooperative

Alex Kallen, MD (infectious disease), Centers for Disease Control

Barnett Kramer, MD (oncology), National Cancer Institute

Leslie (bibliophile/barista), Bozeman Deaconess Hospital

Ana Mata-Fink, MD (orthopedics), Dartmouth-Hitchcock Medical Center

Michael Mayor, MD (orthopedics), Thayer School of Engineering at Dartmouth

David Nierenberg, MD (clinical pharmacology), Dartmouth-Hitchcock Medical Center

Douglas Robertson, MD (gastroenterology), White River Junction VA Medical Center

Kenneth Rosenfield, MD (cardiology), Massachusetts General Hospital

Barry Stults, MD (general internal medicine), University of Utah

E. Donnall Thomas Jr., MD (general internal medicine), Lewistown, Montana

Jean-Paul Toussaint (medical student), University of Washington–Montana
    WWAMI (Washington, Wyoming, Alaska, Montana, and Idaho)

Steven Tower, MD (orthopedics), Providence Alaska Medical Center

Chris Trimble (business administration), Tuck School of Business

Don Trunkey, MD (trauma surgery), Oregon Health Sciences University

James Weinstein, DO, MS (orthopedics), Dartmouth-Hitchcock Medical
    Center

Noel Weiss, MD (epidemiology), University of Washington

NOTES

A NOTE FOR THE academic community (who are likely to be among the few to read this page): This book is purposely meant to be more informal—read: less "scientific"—than my prior books. As part of an effort to communicate more broadly, it is designed to be more accessible to the general public: more narrative, with fewer numbers, and, perhaps most important, no scary tabular and graphical data and no superscript references.

These notes provide interested readers with references to the medical literature used in this book. They may—or may not—be central to the general premise. I particularly wanted to give credit to some of the "classic" observational studies and randomized trials. In addition, I include a few notes pointing to contributions outside of the medical literature that may be of interest.

INTRODUCTION

nearly one-half said their patients received too much medical care B. E. Sirovich et al., "Too Little? Too Much? Primary Care Physicians' Views on US Health Care," *Archives of Internal Medicine* 171, no. 17 (September 26, 2011): 1582–85.

ASSUMPTION #1: ALL RISKS CAN BE LOWERED

in the 1950s, most Massachusetts physicians were smokers L. S. Snegireff and O. M. Lombard, "Survey of Smoking Habits of Massachusetts Physicians," *New England Journal of Medicine* 250, no. 24 (June 17, 1954): 1042–45.

Pittsburgh was the poster child for bad air quality Smoke Control Lantern
   Slide Collection, http://digital.library.pitt.edu/images/pittsburgh
   /smokecontrol.html.

Doll and Hill's stroke of genius: study the physicians themselves Richard
   Doll and A. Bradford Hill, "Lung Cancer and Other Causes of Death in
   Relation to Smoking; A Second Report on the Mortality of British Doc-
   tors," *British Medical Journal* 2, no. 5001 (November 10, 1956): 1071–81.

cancer risk increases with height G. C. Kabat et al., "Adult Stature and Risk
   of Cancer at Different Anatomic Sites in a Cohort of Postmenopausal
   Women," *Cancer Epidemiology, Biomarkers, and Prevention* 22, no. 8
   (August 2013): 1353–63.

short stature is associated with coronary artery disease T. A. Paajanen et al.,
   "Short Stature Is Associated with Coronary Heart Disease: A Systematic
   Review of the Literature and a Meta-Analysis," *European Heart Journal* 31,
   no. 14 (July 2010): 1802–9.

chance happens: astrological signs and hospital admissions P. C. Austin et
   al., "Testing Multiple Statistical Hypotheses Resulted in Spurious Associations: A Study of Astrological Signs and Health," *Journal of Clinical
   Epidemiology* 59, no. 9 (September 2006): 964–69.

the Hill criteria for causation Austin Bradford Hill, "The Environment and
   Disease: Association or Causation?," *Proceedings of the Royal Society of
   Medicine* 58, no. 5 (1965): 295–300.

summary of the evidence for hormone replacement in 1991 E. Barrett-
   Connor and T. L. Bush, "Estrogen and Coronary Heart Disease in
   Women," *Journal of the American Medical Association* 265, no. 14 (April
   10, 1991): 1861–67.

a computer model designed to estimate the effect of hormone replacement
   N. F. Col et al., "Patient-Specific Decisions about Hormone Replacement
   Therapy in Postmenopausal Women," *Journal of the American Medical
   Association* 277, no. 14 (April 9, 1997): 1140–47.

randomized trials of hormone replacement therapy S. Hulley et al., "Randomized Trial of Estrogen Plus Progestin for Secondary Prevention of

Coronary Heart Disease in Postmenopausal Women," *Journal of the American Medical Association* 280, no. 7 (August 19, 1998): 605–13. J. E. Rossouw et al., "Risks and Benefits of Estrogen Plus Progestin in Healthy Postmenopausal Women: Principal Results from the Women's Health Initiative Randomized Controlled Trial," *Journal of the American Medical Association* 288, no. 3 (July 17, 2002): 321–33.

prevention bias D. B. Petitti, "Hormone Replacement Therapy and Heart Disease Prevention: Experimentation Trumps Observation," *Journal of the American Medical Association* 280, no. 7 (August 19, 1998): 650–52.

people interested in screening tend to be healthy P. F. Pinsky et al., "Evidence of a Healthy Volunteer Effect in the Prostate, Lung, Colorectal, and Ovarian Cancer Screening Trial," *American Journal of Epidemiology* 165, no. 8 (April 15, 2007): 874–81.

Framingham Heart Study See "History," http://www.framinghamheartstudy .org/about-fhs/history.php, and "Research Milestones," http://www .framinghamheartstudy.org/about-fhs/research-milestones.php.

VA Cooperative Study of men with really, really high blood pressure Veterans Administration Cooperative Study Group on Antihypertensive Agents, "Effects of Treatment on Morbidity in Hypertension: Results in Patients with Diastolic Blood Pressures Averaging 115 through 129 mm Hg," *Journal of the American Medical Association* 202, no. 11 (December 11, 1967): 1028–34.

left half of the U-shaped curve for blood pressure R. M. Cooper-DeHoff et al., "Tight Blood Pressure Control and Cardiovascular Outcomes among Hypertensive Patients with Diabetes and Coronary Artery Disease," *Journal of the American Medical Association* 304, no. 1 (July 7, 2010): 61–68.

VA study showing blood pressure overtreatment now more common than undertreatment VA Diabetes Quality Enhancement Research Initiative (QUERI) Workgroup on Clinical Action Measures, "Monitoring Performance for Blood Pressure Management among Patients with Diabetes Mellitus: Too Much of a Good Thing?," *Archives of Internal Medicine* 172, no. 12 (June 25, 2012): 938–45.

left half of the U-shaped curve for blood sugar Action to Control Cardiovascular Risk in Diabetes Study Group, "Effects of Intensive Glucose

Lowering in Type 2 Diabetes," *New England Journal of Medicine* 358, no. 24 (June 12, 2008): 2545–59.

regular aspirin for male doctors "Physicians' Health Study: Aspirin and Primary Prevention of Coronary Heart Disease," letter to the editor, *New England Journal of Medicine* 321, no. 26 (December 28, 1989): 1825–28.

Body Mass Index (BMI), another U-shaped curve K. M. Flegal et al., "Association of All-Cause Mortality with Overweight and Obesity Using Standard Body Mass Index Categories: A Systematic Review and Meta-Analysis," *Journal of the American Medical Association* 309, no. 1 (January 2, 2013): 71–82.

ASSUMPTION #2: IT'S ALWAYS BETTER TO FIX THE PROBLEM

Lancet *meta-analysis of angioplasty versus medical management for heart attack* E. C. Keeley et al., "Primary Angioplasty versus Intravenous Thrombolytic Therapy for Acute Myocardial Infarction: A Quantitative Review of 23 Randomised Trials," *Lancet* 361, no. 9351 (January 4, 2003): 13–20.

COURAGE *trial of angioplasty versus medical management for stable angina* W. E. Boden et al.; COURAGE Trial Research Group, "Optimal Medical Therapy with or without PCI for Stable Coronary Disease," *New England Journal of Medicine* 356, no. 15 (April 12, 2007): 1503–16. W. S. Weintraub et al.; COURAGE Trial Research Group, "Effect of PCI on Quality of Life in Patients with Stable Coronary Disease," *New England Journal of Medicine* 359, no. 7 (August 14, 2008): 677–87.

COURAGE *editorial* E. D. Peterson and J. S. Rumsfeld, "Finding the Courage to Reconsider Medical Therapy for Stable Angina," *New England Journal of Medicine* 359, no. 7 (August 14, 2008): 751–53.

fix *versus* manage *strategy for atrial fibrillation—US trial* D. G. Wyse et al.; Atrial Fibrillation Follow-up Investigation of Rhythm Management (AFFIRM) Investigators, "A Comparison of Rate Control and Rhythm Control in Patients with Atrial Fibrillation," *New England Journal of Medicine* 347, no. 23 (December 5, 2002): 1825–33.

fix *versus* manage *strategy for atrial fibrillation—European trial* I. C. Van Gelder et al.; Rate Control versus Electrical Cardioversion for Persistent

Atrial Fibrillation Study Group, "A Comparison of Rate Control and Rhythm Control in Patients with Recurrent Persistent Atrial Fibrillation," *New England Journal of Medicine* 347, no. 23 (December 5, 2002): 1834–40.

ablation complications—Hopkins H. Hoyt et al., "Complications Arising from Catheter Ablation of Atrial Fibrillation: Temporal Trends and Predictors," *Heart Rhythm* 8, no. 12 (December 2011): 1869–74.

ablation complications—Harvard M. Bohnen et al., "Incidence and Predictors of Major Complications from Contemporary Catheter Ablation to Treat Cardiac Arrhythmias," *Heart Rhythm* 8, no. 11 (November 2011): 1661–66.

British Medical Journal parachute parody of evidence-based medicine G. C. Smith and J. P. Pell, "Parachute Use to Prevent Death and Major Trauma Related to Gravitational Challenge: Systematic Review of Randomised Controlled Trials," *British Medical Journal* 327, no. 7429 (December 29, 2003): 1459–61.

ASSUMPTION #3: SOONER IS ALWAYS BETTER

despite three decades of widespread screening mammography in the United States, the rate at which women present with metastatic breast cancer is unchanged A. Bleyer and H. G. Welch, "Effect of Three Decades of Screening Mammography on Breast-Cancer Incidence," *New England Journal of Medicine* 367, no. 21 (November 22, 2012): 1998–2005.

two trials of prostate cancer screening F. H. Schröder et al.; ERSPC Investigators, "Screening and Prostate-Cancer Mortality in a Randomized European Study," *New England Journal of Medicine* 360, no. 13 (March 26, 2009): 1320–28. G. L. Andriole et al.; PLCO Project Team, "Mortality Results from a Randomized Prostate-Cancer Screening Trial," *New England Journal of Medicine* 360, no. 13 (March 26, 2009): 1310–19.

details of the trials of screening mammography H. Gilbert Welch, "Understand the Limits to Research," chapter 9 in Welch, *Should I Be Tested for Cancer? Maybe Not and Here's Why* (Oakland: University of California Press, 2004).

lung cancer screening in heavy smokers National Lung Screening Trial Research Team, "Reduced Lung-Cancer Mortality with Low-Dose Computed Tomographic Screening," *New England Journal of Medicine* 365, no. 5 (August 4, 2011): 395–409.

fecal occult blood screening for colon cancer J. S. Mandel et al.; Minnesota Colon Cancer Control Study, "Reducing Mortality from Colorectal Cancer by Screening for Fecal Occult Blood," *New England Journal of Medicine* 328, no. 19 (May 13, 1993): 1365–71. J. D. Hardcastle et al., "Randomised Controlled Trial of Faecal-Occult-Blood Screening for Colorectal Cancer," *Lancet* 348, no. 9040 (November 30, 1996): 1472–77. E. Lindholm et al., "Survival Benefit in a Randomized Clinical Trial of Faecal Occult Blood Screening for Colorectal Cancer," *British Journal of Surgery* 95, no. 8 (August 2008): 1029–36.

liver and ovarian cancer screening—no effect J. G. Chen et al., "Screening for Liver Cancer: Results of a Randomised Controlled Trial in Qidong, China," *Journal of Medical Screening* 10, no. 4 (2003): 204–9. S. S. Buys et al.; PLCO Project Team, "Effect of Screening on Ovarian Cancer Mortality: The Prostate, Lung, Colorectal and Ovarian (PLCO) Cancer Screening Randomized Controlled Trial," *Journal of the American Medical Association* 305, no. 22 (June 8, 2011): 2295–303.

colon cancer screening—no effect on overall mortality A. Shaukat et al., "Long-Term Mortality after Screening for Colorectal Cancer," *New England Journal of Medicine* 369, no. 12 (September 19, 2013): 1106–14.

easy to see the effect of treatment on overall mortality—the addition of chemotherapy and hormonal therapy to surgery in breast cancer Early Breast Cancer Trialists' Collaborative Group, "Effects of Chemotherapy and Hormonal Therapy for Early Breast Cancer on Recurrence and 15-Year Survival: An Overview of the Randomised Trials," *Lancet* 365, no. 9472 (May 14–20, 2005): 1687–717.

thirty-day mortality rate from mastectomy is about a quarter of 1 percent M. B. El-Tamer et al., "Morbidity and Mortality Following Breast Cancer Surgery in Women: National Benchmarks for Standards of Care," *Annals of Surgery* 245, no. 5 (May 2007): 665–71.

false alarms from screening mammography—data from the mammographers themselves R. A. Hubbard et al., "Cumulative Probability of False-Positive Recall or Biopsy Recommendation after 10 Years of Screening Mammography: A Cohort Study," *Annals of Internal Medicine* 155, no. 8 (October 18, 2011): 481–92.

false alarms from screening mammography—psychological effects J. Brodersen and V. D. Siersma, "Long-Term Psychosocial Consequences of False-Positive Screening Mammography," *Annals of Family Medicine* 11, no. 2 (March–April 2013): 106–15.

Dr. Crile in Life *magazine 1955* George Crile Jr., "A Plea Against the Blind Fear of Cancer: An Experienced Surgeon Says That Excessive Worry Leads to Costly Tests, Undue Suffering and Unnecessary Operations," *Life*, October 31, 1955, 128–42.

thirty-day mortality rate from prostatectomy is about a half of 1 percent S. M. Alibhai et al., "30-Day Mortality and Major Complications after Radical Prostatectomy: Influence of Age and Comorbidity," *Journal of the National Cancer Institute* 97, no. 20 (October 19, 2005): 1525–32. J. J. Liu et al., "Perioperative Outcomes for Laparoscopic and Robotic Compared with Open Prostatectomy Using the National Surgical Quality Improvement Program (NSQIP) Database," *Urology* 82, no. 3 (September 2013): 579–83.

overdiagnosis prostate cancer screening—over a million American men H. G. Welch and P. C. Albertsen, "Prostate Cancer Diagnosis and Treatment after the Introduction of Prostate-Specific Antigen Screening: 1986-2005," *Journal of the National Cancer Institute* 101, no. 19 (October 7, 2009): 1325–29.

overdiagnosis breast cancer screening—over a million American women A. Bleyer and H. G. Welch, "Effect of Three Decades of Screening Mammography on Breast-Cancer Incidence," *New England Journal of Medicine* 367, no. 21 (November 22, 2012): 1998–2005.

overdiagnosis, other harms—suicide F. Fang et al., "Suicide and Cardiovascular Death after a Cancer Diagnosis," *New England Journal of Medicine* 366, no. 14 (April 5, 2012): 1310–18.

overdiagnosis, other harms—bankruptcy S. Ramsey et al., "Washington State Cancer Patients Found to Be at Greater Risk for Bankruptcy Than People Without a Cancer Diagnosis," *Health Affairs* 32, no. 6 (June 2013): 1143–52.

UK National Health Service mammography screening pamphlet NHS *Breast Screening: Helping You Decide* (London: Academic Health Sciences Centre, June 2013), http://www.cancerscreening.nhs.uk/breastscreen /publications/nhsbsp.pdf.

David Smithers: "Cancer is no more a disease of cells" D. W. Smithers, "An Attack on Cytologism," *Lancet* 1, no. 7228 (March 10, 1962): 493–99.

ASSUMPTION #4: IT NEVER HURTS TO GET MORE INFORMATION

effect of more information—enhanced communication in primary care M. Weinberger et al.; Veterans Affairs Cooperative Study Group on Primary Care and Hospital Readmission, "Does Increased Access to Primary Care Reduce Hospital Readmissions?," *New England Journal of Medicine* 334, no. 22 (May 30, 1996): 1441–47.

effect of more information—lung impedance in congestive heart failure patients D. J. van Veldhuisen et al.; DOT-HF Investigators, "Intrathoracic Impedance Monitoring, Audible Patient Alerts, and Outcome in Patients with Heart Failure," *Circulation* 124, no. 16 (October 18, 2011): 1719–26. J. E. Udelson, "T.M.I. (Too Much Information)?," *Circulation* 124, no. 16 (October 18, 2011): 1697–99.

effect of more information—surveillance for metastases in breast cancer patients M. Rosselli Del Turco et al., "Intensive Diagnostic Follow-Up after Treatment of Primary Breast Cancer: A Randomized Trial; National Research Council Project on Breast Cancer Follow-Up," *Journal of the American Medical Association* 271, no. 20 (May 25, 1994): 1593–97. GIVIO Investigators, "Impact of Follow-Up Testing on Survival and Health-Related Quality of Life in Breast Cancer Patients: A Multicenter Randomized Controlled Trial," *Journal of the American Medical Association* 271, no. 20 (May 25, 1994): 1587–92.

effect of more information—surveillance for metastases in colon cancer patients John N. Primrose et al., "Effect of 3 to 5 Years of Scheduled CEA and CT Follow-Up to Detect Recurrence of Colorectal Cancer: The FACS Randomized Clinical Trial," *Journal of the American Medical Association* 311, no. 3 (January 15, 2014): 263–70.

data, information, useful knowledge—Ken Ringle in the **Washington Post** Ken Ringle, "When More Is Less; The Smithsonian's Dazzling, Orwellian 'Information Age,'" *Washington Post*, May 6, 1990, http://www.highbeam .com/doc/1P2-1125285.html.

home glucose monitoring led to more distress and depression M. Franciosi et al.; Qualita' ed Esito in Diabetologia (QuED) Project, "The Impact of Blood Glucose Self-Monitoring on Metabolic Control and Quality of Life in Type 2 Diabetic Patients: An Urgent Need for Better Educational Strategies," *Diabetes Care* 24, no. 11 (November 2001): 1870–77.

VA Cooperative Study of men with really, really high blood pressure Veterans Administration Cooperative Study Group on Antihypertensive Agents, "Effects of Treatment on Morbidity in Hypertension: Results in Patients with Diastolic Blood Pressures Averaging 115 Through 129 mm Hg," *Journal of the American Medical Association* 202, no. 11 (December 11, 1967): 1028–34.

the cascade effect J. W. Mold and H. F. Stein, "The Cascade Effect in the Clinical Care of Patients," *New England Journal of Medicine* 314, no. 8 (February 20, 1986): 512–14.

ASSUMPTION #5: ACTION IS ALWAYS BETTER THAN INACTION

medical care for our four assassinated presidents D. Trunkey and F. Farjah, "Medical and Surgical Care of our Four Assassinated Presidents," *Journal of the American College of Surgeons* 201, no. 6 (December 2005): 976–89.

as late as 1882 "anti-Listerians" were in the majority G. T. Wrench, *Lord Lister: His Life and Work* (London: T. Fisher Unwin, 1914), 263–64.

adherence to hand washing recommendations in the hospital less than 50 percent V. Erasmus et al., "Systematic Review of Studies on Compliance with Hand Hygiene Guidelines in Hospital Care," *Infection Control and Hospital Epidemiology* 31, no. 3 (March 2010): 283–94.

CDC estimate of the number of deaths associated with health care–associated infections R. M. Klevens et al., "Estimating Health Care–Associated Infections and Deaths in US Hospitals, 2002," *Public Health Reports* 122, no. 2 (March–April 2007): 160–66.

recommendations regarding prophylactic wisdom teeth extractions NICE (National Institute for Health and Care Excellence), *Guidance on the Extraction of Wisdom Teeth* (London: National Institute for Clinical Excellence, March 2000), http://www.nice.org.uk/nicemedia/live/11385 /31993/31993.pdf. American Public Health Association, "Opposition to Prophylactic Removal of Third Molars (Wisdom Teeth)," policy statement, October 28, 2008, http://www.apha.org/advocacy/policy/policysearch /default.htm?id=1371.

postoperative cognitive dysfunction J. T. Moller et al.; International Study of Post-Operative Cognitive Dysfunction, "Long-Term Postoperative Cognitive Dysfunction in the Elderly ISPOCD1 Study," *Lancet* 351, no. 9106 (March 21, 1998): 857–61.

back surgery for work-related back pain in Ohio T. H. Nguyen et al., "Long-Term Outcomes of Lumbar Fusion among Workers' Compensation Subjects: A Historical Cohort Study," *Spine* 36, no. 4 (February 15, 2011): 320–31.

neurosurgeon reports 14 percent of patients scheduled for back surgery have no abnormality N. E. Epstein and D. C. Hood, "'Unnecessary' Spinal Surgery: A Prospective 1-Year Study of One Surgeon's Experience," *Surgical Neurology International* 2, no. 83 (June 21, 2011), doi: 10.4103/2152-7806.82249.

back surgery is all over the map *Spine Surgery: A Report by the Dartmouth Atlas of Health Care* (Lebanon, NH: Center for the Evaluative Clinical Sciences, 2006), http://www.dartmouthatlas.org/downloads/reports /Spine_Surgery_2006.pdf.

federal agency evaluating medical care threatened by spine surgeons B. H. Gray et al., "AHCPR and the Changing Politics of Health Services Research," *Health Affairs*, supplementary web exclusives (January–June 2003): W3-283-307.

effect of minimally invasive gall bladder surgery on volume of surgery and the number of deaths C. A. Steiner et al., "Surgical Rates and Operative Mortality for Open and Laparoscopic Cholecystectomy in Maryland," *New England Journal of Medicine* 330, no. 6 (February 10, 1994): 403–8.

four randomized trials of knee arthroscopy in patients with arthritis J. B. Moseley et al., "A Controlled Trial of Arthroscopic Surgery for Osteoarthritis of the Knee," *New England Journal of Medicine* 347, no. 2 (July 11, 2002): 81–88. A. Kirkley et al., "A Randomized Trial of Arthroscopic Surgery for Osteoarthritis of the Knee," *New England Journal of Medicine* 359, no. 11 (September 11, 2008): 1097–107. J. N. Katz et al., "Surgery versus Physical Therapy for a Meniscal Tear and Osteoarthritis," *New England Journal of Medicine* 368, no. 18 (May 2, 2013): 1675–84. R. Sihvonen et al.; Finnish Degenerative Meniscal Lesion Study Group, "Arthroscopic Partial Meniscectomy versus Sham Surgery for a Degenerative Meniscal Tear," *New England Journal of Medicine* 369, no. 26 (December 26, 2013): 2515–24.

ASSUMPTION #6: NEWER IS ALWAYS BETTER

Vioxx causes heart attacks and strokes R. S. Bresalier et al.; Adenomatous Polyp Prevention on Vioxx Trial Investigators, "Cardiovascular Events Associated with Rofecoxib in a Colorectal Adenoma Chemoprevention Trial," *New England Journal of Medicine* 352, no. 11 (March 17, 2005): 1092–102.

bone marrow transplantation for metastatic breast cancer—the story H. G. Welch and J. Mogielnicki, "Presumed Benefit: Lessons from the American Experience with Marrow Transplantation for Breast Cancer," *British Medical Journal* 324, no. 7345 (May 4, 2002): 1088–92.

bone marrow transplantation for metastatic breast cancer—the trial E. A. Stadtmauer et al.; Philadelphia Bone Marrow Transplant Group, "Conventional-Dose Chemotherapy Compared with High-Dose Chemotherapy Plus Autologous Hematopoietic Stem-Cell Transplantation for Metastatic Breast Cancer," *New England Journal of Medicine* 342, no. 15 (April 13, 2000): 1069–76.

bone marrow transplantation for metastatic breast cancer—the editorial
M. E. Lippman, "High-Dose Chemotherapy Plus Autologous Bone Marrow Transplantation for Metastatic Breast Cancer," *New England Journal of Medicine* 342, no. 15 (April 13, 2000): 1119–20.

bone marrow transplantation for metastatic breast cancer—the 2011 overview D. A. Berry et al., "High-Dose Chemotherapy with Autologous Hematopoietic Stem-Cell Transplantation in Metastatic Breast Cancer: Overview of Six Randomized Trials," *Journal of Clinical Oncology* 29, no. 24 (August 20, 2011): 3224–31.

concern about quality in new, low volume centers performing bone marrow transplantation C. S. Chen et al., "Safeguarding the Administration of High-Dose Chemotherapy: A National Practice Survey by the American Society for Blood and Marrow Transplantation," *Biology of Blood and Marrow Transplantation* 3, no. 6 (December 1997): 331–40.

payments to orthopedic surgeons J. M. Hockenberry et al., "Financial Payments by Orthopedic Device Makers to Orthopedic Surgeons," *Archives of Internal Medicine* 171, no. 19 (October 24, 2011): 1759–65.

case reports of cobalt poisoning following hip replacement K. Dahms et al., "Cobalt Intoxication Diagnosed with the Help of Dr. House," *Lancet* 383, no. 9916 (February 8, 2014): 574. L. A. Allen et al., "Clinical Problem-Solving: Missing Elements of the History," *New England Journal of Medicine* 370, no. 6 (February 6, 2014): 559–66.

mini-epidemics of cobalt poisoning in Quebec and Omaha G. Mercier and G. Patry, "Quebec Beer-Drinkers' Cardiomyopathy: Clinical Signs and Symptoms," *Canadian Medical Association Journal* 97, no. 15 (October 7, 1967): 884–88. P. H. McDermott et al., "Myocardosis and Cardiac Failure in Men," *Journal of the American Medical Association* 198, no. 3 (October 17, 1966): 253–56.

metal on metal implants five times more likely to fail National Joint Registry for England, Wales, and Northern Ireland, *Tenth Annual Report 2013*, http://www.njrcentre.org.uk/njrcentre/default.aspx.

Mayo Clinic experience from 1970 D. J. Berry et al., "Twenty-Five-Year Survivorship of Two Thousand Consecutive Primary Charnley Total Hip Replacements: Factors Affecting Survivorship of Acetabular and Femoral Components," *Journal of Bone and Joint Surgery* 84–A, no. 2 (February 2002): 171–77.

ASSUMPTION #7: IT'S ALL ABOUT AVOIDING DEATH

preferences about receiving chemotherapy in patients with advanced lung cancer G. Silvestri et al., "Preferences for Chemotherapy in Patients with Advanced Non-Small Cell Lung Cancer: Descriptive Study Based on Scripted Interviews," *British Medical Journal* 317, no. 7161 (September 19, 1998): 771–75.

care at the end of life in "America's Best Hospitals" J. E. Wennberg et al., "Use of Hospitals, Physician Visits, and Hospice Care During Last Six Months of Life Among Cohorts Loyal to Highly Respected Hospitals in the United States," *British Medical Journal* 328, no. 7440 (March 13, 2004): 607.

preferences for local versus regional surgery S. R. Finlayson et al., "Patient Preferences for Location of Care: Implications for Regionalization," *Medical Care* 37, no. 2 (February 1999): 204–9.

live longer with palliative care J. S. Temel et al., "Early Palliative Care for Patients with Metastatic Non-Small-Cell Lung Cancer," *New England Journal of Medicine* 363, no. 8 (August 19, 2010): 733–42.

CONCLUSION

defining health M. Huber et al., "How Should We Define Health?," *British Medical Journal* 343 (July 26, 2011): d4163.

income and social status—Whitehall Study M. G. Marmot et al., "Inequalities in Death—Specific Explanations of a General Pattern?," *Lancet* 1, no. 8384 (May 5, 1984): 1003–6.

providing support may be more important to health than receiving it S. G. Post, "Altruism, Happiness, and Health: It's Good to Be Good," *International Journal of Behavioral Medicine* 12, no. 2 (2005): 66–77.

INDEX